NATURAL REMEDIES *for a* HEALTHY HEART

DAVID HEBER, M.D., Ph.D.

Avery Publishing Group
Garden City Park, New York

The medical information and procedures contained in this book are based upon the research, and personal and professional experiences, of the author. The author and the publisher do not advocate the use of any particular form of health care but believe that the information presented in this book should be available to the public. This book is not intended to replace the advice and treatment of a physician. Any use of the information set forth herein is entirely at the reader's discretion.

Because there is always some risk involved, the author and the publisher are not responsible for any adverse effects or consequences resulting from the use of any of the preparations or procedures in this book. Please do not use this book if you are unwilling to assume the risk. Each person and situation are unique, and a physician or other qualified health professional should be consulted if there is any question regarding the presence or treatment of any abnormal health condition. It is a sign of wisdom, not cowardice, to seek a second or third opinion.

Cover design:
William Gonzalez and
  Rudy Shur
Typesetter: Al Berotti
In-house editor: Lisa James

Avery Publishing Group, Inc.
120 Old Broadway
Garden City Park, New York 11040
1-800-548-5757

Cataloging-in-Publication Data

Heber, David
    Natural remedies for a healthy heart : remarkable breakthroughs for lowering cholesterol, lessening blood pressure, and reversing cardiovascular disease / David Heber.
    p. cm.
    Includes bibliographical references and index.
    ISBN: 0-89529-808-2

    1. Heart—Diseases—Diet therapy. 2. Cardiovascular pharmacology. 3. Stress management. I. Title.

RC684.D5H43   1998   616.1'2'06
                                    QBI97-40768

Printed in the United States of America

10 9 8 7 6 5 4 3 2 1

Contents

Dedicated to Mr. Ray Stark,
whose interest in healthy nutrition
and dietary supplements
inspired me to vigorously pursue
the research described in this book

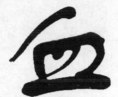

Blood

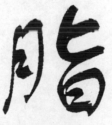

Fat

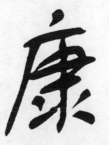

Healthy or Happy

Acknowledgments

I would like to acknowledge Dr. David Kritchevsky of the Wistar Institute in Philadelphia, who is also an Adjunct Professor at UCLA, for reviewing this manuscript for accuracy. His great knowledge of this field and fine sense of humor are an inspiration to everyone working in the field of nutrition. I would also like to thank Dr. Bill Go and Dr. Judith Ashley, who have reviewed the manuscript based on their extensive experience in human nutrition. A very special thanks goes to Mr. Dave Tuttle, who helped to develop this manuscript and kept me on target until its completion. Finally, I would like to thank my wife, Anita, who put up with my long periods of preoccupation and computer punching while I completed this manuscript.

Preface

As we move into the next millennium, we are constantly reminded how technology is changing our lives. Nowhere is this more evident than in modern-day medicine. Yet we are coming to realize that there is a downside to these advances.

I have been working in the field of preventive medicine for the last twenty years as a physician specializing in internal medicine, endocrinology, and metabolism. As one of only about 300 American physicians certified in nutrition, I have also been doing basic and clinical research on nutrition and prevention, using both my medical training and my doctorate in physiology. I have been in the unique position of having one foot in the highly technical world of laboratory research and the other in the clinical world of patients and patient-based research. This has increased my understanding of the cellular basis of chronic disease while giving me insight into what motivates people to change their behavior in heart-healthy ways.

I have begun to appreciate the power of natural therapies to prevent heart disease and other chronic diseases. The healing power of herbs has been known for centuries, but while most of my patients have been interested in these approaches, they have felt that they were somewhat mysterious and quite possibly dangerous. In the research I have done for this book, I have relied on established principles of biology and medicine. The natural medicines I will discuss have been tested, and been found to be safe and effective.

Every drug has certain side effects. When curing disease, these side effects are usually worth the risk involved, since the benefit of the drug outweighs the downside of the side effects experienced. Yet this argument breaks down when applied to prevention. In otherwise healthy people who have moderately high cholesterol levels, the side effects of these drugs can become a major problem. The costs and side effects associated with these medicines just don't make sense.

In searching for a better way, I have discovered that not everyone can achieve an appropriate reduction in cholesterol levels through diet alone. Even diet combined with exercise and stress reduction may not be enough to effectively lower cholesterol levels in everyone. Is there something beyond diet, and less expensive and risky than prescription drugs that can be used to prevent heart disease?

Yes, there is. Recent research has shown that there are a number of effective natural therapies that will lower your cholesterol level and reduce your risk of heart disease. These natural products, including garlic, phytosterols, aspirin, niacin, antioxidants, fiber, and a new dietary supplement called Cholestin-3, can improve the health of both your heart and your entire cardiovascular system.

In this book, I have put these new products into perspective by including recommendations on diet, exercise, and stress reduction. I have brought this together into a plan that you can implement with the help and approval of your doctor. After numerous conversations with my colleagues, I believe there is widespread support for this natural approach to prevention.

Among the millions of Americans who have heart-disease risk factors such as high cholesterol, obesity, smoking, high blood pressure, diabetes, or an unfavorable family history, prevention makes great sense. This book will benefit those who already have heart disease, but it is mostly directed at their families, friends, and neighbors—and you! This book also has implications for other diseases of aging, including common forms of cancer such as breast cancer, prostate cancer, and colon cancer. Studies show that the same countries that have a high incidence of heart disease also have high incidences of these forms of cancer.

Natural remedies have a long tradition of use, but they are not the medicines of the past. As we combine our modern understanding of chronic disease with an examination of these natural remedies, we find something very interesting. Rather than being pure single substances, as many modern medicines are, natural remedies are often complex mixtures of several different substances that work in combination. Many modern drugs are derived from plant sources. When these drugs are prepared, they are separated from the natural environment of antioxidants and other chemicals that occur naturally in plants. It is conceivable that these other substances, which are thought of as "impurities" by the drug companies, might actually help natural remedies work better with fewer side effects.

I plan to spend the rest of my professional career investigating the actions of natural remedies in the context of a healthy diet and lifestyle. I think this work can make a world of difference for you and your heart. Let *Natural Remedies for a Healthy Heart* be your guide.

CHAPTER 1

The New Path to a Healthy Heart

I f you have picked up this book, chances are that you are concerned about high cholesterol levels and heart disease. In this book, you will discover a new path to a healthy heart that is natural and more powerful than that of the most advanced and expensive prescription drugs. For many people with high cholesterol, diet is not enough. If you are one of those people, your doctor may have suggested that you use a cholesterol-lowering medication. These drugs can be costly and are sometimes associated with side effects. Is there a more natural way for you to lower your cholesterol level safely and effectively?

Yes. A new scientific understanding of heart disease has pointed the way to natural therapies. Research over the past twenty years in the field of prevention has demonstrated the power of diet, exercise, and stress reduction. Recently, a number of plant- and yeast-derived natural therapies have also been tested and found effective. I will review the scientific findings of studies conducted in the last few years and put this information into perspective as part of an overall program designed to lower your cholesterol level. You and your physician will then be able to put this knowledge to work for you.

Perhaps you already have heart disease and would like to know what you can do to reverse the changes taking place in your heart. There is some exciting new information in this book on how you can reverse some of that damage and prevent any further damage to this vital organ. I have been studying this subject for over twenty years, and the last few have been the most exciting. I will not only tell you about heart disease, but will explain in clear, simple language what you can do about it.

If you are already being treated for heart disease or a high cholesterol level, please be sure to check with your doctor before making any changes in diet or medication. I believe you will find increasing support among physicians for healthy preventive strategies, and I am working to convince more physicians of the power of prevention. Now, let's preview what this book will cover by answering some important questions.

DOESN'T HEART DISEASE HAPPEN SUDDENLY?

No. Heart disease begins early in life. Over time, cholesterol is deposited on the walls of the heart's blood vessels. It is easier to reverse the effects of heart disease in the earliest stages, when the blood vessel walls contain relatively small amounts of cholesterol. As time goes on, cholesterol is chemically changed by various waste products in the walls of the blood vessel. This results in more cholesterol being trapped. This modified cholesterol attracts white blood cells that try to clean up the buildup of foreign material but in the process do even more damage. Then real bone forms in the vessel walls. By the time your arteries have hardened, you actually have thin sheaths of bone all around the blood vessel wall. This process progresses over many decades.

A heart attack doesn't happen until a clot forms in the narrowed blood vessel, and blocks the blood flow entirely. If this blockage is discovered immediately, doctors can give you an intravenous injection of enzymes that chew up the clot. This will often limit or eliminate significant damage to your heart. Doctors will sometimes recommend angioplasty as well, in which a stainless steel mesh called a stent is placed in the area of blockage to provide an artificial channel for blood flow. Some patients have such a high degree of blockage that a bypass operation is needed. During this operation, veins from the legs are stitched into the coronary vessels on the surface of the heart to carry blood around the obstructed areas. While you have a good chance of surviving such an ordeal with the help of modern medicine, I will explain how to prevent heart disease and reverse its effects naturally. There is a lot you can do right now. For more information on the heart itself, see Chapter 2.

HOW HIGH IS A "HIGH" CHOLESTEROL LEVEL?

The answer to this question depends on where you live in the world. In some countries, our average cholesterol level would be considered high. But even in the United States, our average cholesterol levels have dropped as we have improved our diets and lifestyle. Some experts believe that when your cholesterol is low enough (less than 160 milligrams per deciliter, or mg/dL), the process of atherosclerosis stops and may even go into reverse. Everyone has a characteristic cholesterol level that is a result of their genes, diet, and lifestyle. You will learn how to lower your cholesterol level naturally through diet and other natural therapies. For more information on heart-disease rates and risk factors, see Chapter 3.

ISN'T A HIGH CHOLESTEROL LEVEL THE SAME THING AS HEART DISEASE?

No. Cholesterol level is one indication of your risk for heart disease, but there are other risk factors. Cholesterol level has become so identified with heart disease in the public's mind that many people mistakenly think they are one and the same. While cholesterol is one of the most important risk factors, it would be a mistake to ignore the others. In this book, you will discover that many things affect the cholesterol level in your blood. You will find out how your level of cholesterol is controlled by a cholesterol thermostat. You will also learn how natural medicines can act together to reduce cholesterol and reverse the effects of atherosclerosis, or hardening of the arteries. For more information on what determines your cholesterol level, see Chapter 4.

CAN'T I JUST EAT A SLIGHTLY DIFFERENT DIET TO PREVENT HEART DISEASE?

For most people, the answer is no. Obesity is the most common nutritional disorder in the United States, so losing weight is definitely one natural path to a healthy heart. If you are overweight, you may also have high blood pressure as well as high levels of cholesterol and triglycerides (fats). As a result, obesity is perhaps the most common reason for the high level of heart disease in the United States. Most of my patients who are trying to lose weight find it easier to make a big change in diet than a small one. If you stretch a rubber band, it goes back to the same position. If you break a rubber band, it stays broken. I will teach you simple ways to change what you eat and show you how to control the amount you eat. In the future, our food supply may be engineered to provide naturally occurring plant chemicals that will enhance our health. Until then, you will find my diet strategies helpful in your effort to navigate through a high-fat world. Even if you are not overweight, there are many things you can do to maintain a healthy heart by changing the way you eat.

My greatest successes often come with people who are new to nutrition. These newcomers experience the excitement of discovering new knowledge. So if you don't have a lot of prejudices, you are actually ahead of the game. We learn a lot of misinformation about nutrition from food advertising, and then consider it common sense. Albert Einstein once said that common sense is the set of prejudices we acquire by adulthood. My job in this book is to unteach some of these prejudices based on what I have learned about nutrition and heart disease over the past twenty years. For more information on diet, see Chapter 5.

ARE YOU ONE OF THOSE FAD-DIET GURUS WHO IS GOING TO PUT ME ON AN IMPOSSIBLE DIET?

No. I will show you the best ways to eat your way to a healthy heart, but guilt is not a part of this book. Whenever you do something good for your body, so much the better. Now, if you happen to eat a piece of cheese or chocolate cake at a birthday party, don't feel guilty. Put that behind you, and tomorrow start again to control what you eat. Since our foods are often provided to us without our knowing exactly what is in them, it is imperative that we filter what gets past our lips. I will teach you how to filter your diet by reducing or avoiding those foods with lots of fat, while also paying attention to the overall composition of your diet, including protein and sugar.

Consider the wisdom of the Bible. The first dietary guideline in the book of Genesis is to eat the fruits and vegetables of the trees and shrubs. In the book of Exodus, we are told to cut away visible fat. Unfortunately, our ancestors did not anticipate modern agricultural methods for creating high-fat meat products, in which there is fat between the muscle fibers. This modern method considerably reduces the benefit of cutting away visible fat. For more information on the pitfalls of the modern diet, see Chapter 5.

WHAT ABOUT EXERCISE AND STRESS REDUCTION?

Diet alone cannot do everything. It turns out that exercise is a great stress reducer as well as an antidepressant. It can even increase your muscle mass. This gain in muscle mass actually lowers your cholesterol by increasing the activity of certain enzymes that remove cholesterol from the bloodstream. The enlarged muscles also help to pump blood around the body, making your heart's job that much easier. And building muscle will increase your metabolic rate, making you a more effective fat-burning machine and lowering your cholesterol level. It is also important to learn other methods of stress reduction, since stress can harm your health. For more information on stress reduction, see Chapter 6. For more information on exercise, see Chapter 7.

ARE DRUGS REALLY NECESSARY?

Looking beyond diet and lifestyle, I will show you how

to lower your cholesterol using natural therapies rather than drugs. Although about one-quarter of all our drugs were originally derived from plants, these drugs have been chemically processed to remove impurities. However, many of these so-called "impurities" are actually products that Nature included to reduce the side effects of the "active ingredient." For instance, one natural product that you will learn about has a number of related compounds that work together to lower cholesterol by affecting Nature's cholesterol thermostat. One of these natural compounds is found in a pure drug that you can buy. However, the combination of natural cholesterol-lowering substances can lower both cholesterol *and* triglyceride levels. Often it requires a combination of active ingredients to mimic the awesome power of prevention that we can find in Nature. Since you or someone you love may already be taking a prescription cholesterol-lowering drug, I think it is important to discuss such drugs in this book. For more information on this topic, see Chapter 8.

HOW CAN I HARNESS NATURE'S POWER TO KEEP MY HEART HEALTHY?

This book will show you how to harvest Nature's power for disease prevention from among the 10,000 to 50,000 edible species of plants on Earth. Vegetables, fruits, and other plant-derived foods have been on this planet for about a billion years. Modern humans have been here only 50,000 years. That is a mere blink of the eye compared with the plant kingdom.

What can we learn from the plant world? Beyond fruits and vegetables, there is a world of herbs and spices that have the power to reverse abnormal cell growth in the laboratory, and that may have a role in the fight against heart disease and cancer. You will also learn how to harness the power of your body's support systems, such as the nervous and immune systems, and the system of hormone-secreting tissues and organs. By kicking in whenever you do something good for yourself, these defense systems give your body the maximum benefit of healthy changes in lifestyle. So if you are worried about taking drugs, and want to learn how you can take advantage of a number of natural paths to a healthy heart, see Chapters 9 and 10.

WHY DO YOU THINK THAT READING THIS BOOK WILL HELP ME DO ANYTHING FOR MY HEART?

I have written this book based on more than twenty years of research into and observation of the medical and public health strategies for heart disease prevention. I have also helped hundreds of patients change their lifestyles. I learned much of the science I needed soon after I finished my formal education, but I learned how to be a doctor from many years of helping individual patients. In our medical school, we call this art of medicine "doctoring." The word "doctor" originates from the Latin for "teacher." I see this book as an extension of my doctoring activities. For more information on how to combine diet, exercise, stress reduction, and plant-based therapy into a heart-healthy lifestyle, see Chapter 11.

This book is about a new natural path to a healthy heart. It combines the insights of traditional herbal medicine with a modern scientific understanding of the role that cholesterol plays in heart disease and other chronic diseases. I will suggest the use of natural products that contain a number of different substances, substances that work together to produce a gentler lowering of cholesterol levels. I will also suggest a sensible program of diet, exercise, and lifestyle change. You will find that the knowledge in this book will help you to take charge of your health. The end result will be a healthier and richer life free of heart disease.

CHAPTER 2

The Nature of the Human Heart

In fable and myth, the heart is the seat of human emotions. We draw pictures of the heart on Valentine's Day and speak of a broken heart when we lose someone we love. Some people, though, think of the heart as a simple pump. The truth actually lies between these two extremes. Your heart is an integral part of your physical and emotional being. It responds to a variety of stimuli, both good and bad. This new understanding has allowed scientists to discover a number of effective, natural pathways to a healthy heart.

This chapter looks at the intricacies of the heart muscle and how it responds to stress, and gives a basic explanation of what atherosclerosis is and how it occurs. (See Chapter 4 for a detailed explanation of the different types of cholesterol and how they are controlled by what I call the cholesterol thermostat.) Knowledge alone doesn't change behavior, so none of this information is required for you to use the diet, exercise, stress reduction, and natural therapy chapters in the book. However, I think you will find it informative and fascinating.

THE UNIQUE HEART MUSCLE

The heart works together with your muscles to pump blood around your body. How hard it has to work is determined in part by your *blood pressure*. Blood pressure is a measure of the resistance to blood flow in the tiny vessels known as capillaries. The healthy heart beats 100,000 times per day for years on end, keeping its own characteristic rhythm. In seventy years, your heart will beat nearly 2.6 billion times and pump some 35.8 million gallons of blood. It is truly amazing that this biological machine is capable of such uncompromising and faithful work. It far exceeds the productivity of even the most efficient man-made device.

Your heart is divided into two halves, the right and the left. The right half receives the blood returning from every other part of the body after oxygen has been extracted by the various tissues and organs. The right half then pumps this oxygen-deficient blood into your lungs through a vessel called the pulmonary artery. While in the lungs, the blood picks up oxygen, giving it a brighter red hue. The oxygenated blood then flows into the left half of your heart, which pumps the blood out into the *aorta,* the largest artery in the human body. From here, the blood passes into all of the other arteries in your body.

Your heart is connected to your *unconscious nervous system*, also called the autonomic nervous system. This system maintains functions such as temperature control and the movement of food through the intestines. In fact, it is responsible for all of the body's automatic functions, including heartbeat. When you are under stress, your nervous system increases its activity, causing your heart to beat faster. Sometimes this occurs in response to stresses that you can't consciously pinpoint. This mind-body connection can cause your heart to race and can elevate your blood pressure, too. The heart also conditions itself to your usual levels of physical activity and emotional stress.

In order to function, the heart needs a never-ending supply of oxygen. Unlike the other muscles of your body, which can perform physical work in the absence of oxygen, the heart muscle depends on a continuous supply of this vital gas. Therefore, during each beat, the heart also supplies blood to itself, delivering oxygen and other critical nutrients that allow it to maintain its constant pumping action. It is the only organ responsible for providing its own blood supply. This is no mean feat, since the heart needs as much as a pint of blood per minute to sustain its functions. Nearly 5 percent of the blood pumped by the heart goes immediately into the *coronary arteries* to keep the heart beating right on schedule.

Pulsating rhythmically over the heart's moving surface, your coronary arteries and blood vessels work as a team, making sure that every square inch of the surface receives adequate nutrients and oxygen. If one vessel goes into spasm while you're exerting yourself, another vessel opens up more to furnish blood to the undernourished areas of your heart. Over time, these arteries can even grow in order to supply more blood to the heart muscle.

One of the most important reasons the heart needs a continual blood supply is to sustain its electrical activity. The heart is a complex pump that functions much like a solid-state computer chip. Multiple electrical patterns pass over the heart's surface in a rhythmic pattern, directing the proper contraction of the muscles. Every time your heart contracts, nervous impulses are translated into electromagnetic energy waves that travel through the heart's muscle cells. It is this electrical energy that is detected by the electrocardiogram (EKG) taken by your doctor.

THE INCREDIBLY RESILIENT HUMAN HEART

The heart can adjust to many stresses. These include stresses caused by various genetic defects, which can cause some adults to have holes between the chambers of their hearts, or those caused by abnormal valves, which distort the volumes and pressures of the pumping chambers.

Through its complex series of interconnected arteries and veins, the heart is able to redistribute blood flow in response to exertion or stress of most any kind. In general, if one vessel is blocked, the heart can, over time, develop alternate routes to provide blood supply to the undernourished areas of muscle through internal adjustments in blood flow and nervous-system signals. The heart can actually grow new blood vessels, too. It even tries to compensate when parts of its own muscle die from lack of oxygen by causing other areas of the heart muscle to thicken and increase their pumping efficiency. (Recently, surgeons have been cutting out the dead areas of heart muscle in patients with heart failure, which permits the remaining muscle to work more efficiently.)

The heart's adaptability depends on the health of its coronary arteries, which in turn depend on the health of their inner linings. The tissue that lines the inner surfaces of the coronary arteries is called the *endothelium.* However, the endothelium is more than a simple lining. It plays an important role in the development and prevention of heart disease.

A healthy endothelium maintains the normal tone of the blood vessels through its effects on the smooth muscle in the outer part of the vessel wall. The endothelium also plays an important role in controlling the stickiness of *platelets*, which are small cells in the blood. These platelets normally help stop the bleeding when you cut yourself, but they also cling to any tears in the lining of the blood vessels. Thus, they can contribute to the process by which arteries become narrowed and diseased.

In a normal endothelium, a chemical called *acetylcholine* causes the blood vessel to dilate. However, if the endothelium is injured or if there is too much cholesterol in the bloodstream, acetylcholine will cause the vessel to constrict. In other words, even in the absence of heart disease, increased cholesterol levels are associated with abnormal functioning of the heart's blood vessels. Some cholesterol-lowering drugs can restore the ability of the coronary arteries to expand normally in response to acetylcholine. The heart's blood vessels have also been shown to constrict in response to excessive exertion or mental stress, reducing oxygen delivery to the heart. This results in chest pains and could even trigger a heart attack.

All in all, Nature has provided a remarkable system to keep blood flowing to the heart. Through a system of duplicated vessels, every blood vessel has its own backup. The coordination of this marvelous system is under the control of the unconscious nervous system, which regulates the pacemakers in the heart and the complex electromagnetic signals traveling over the surface of the heart. Within each blood vessel, endothelial cells exert their own control.

HOW ARTERIES BECOME CLOGGED

Atherosclerosis, also known as hardening of the arteries, is the complex process by which arteries become narrowed with cholesterol deposits known as *plaques*. (For a more detailed explanation of the role of cholesterol in plaque formation, see Chapter 4.) Recent studies have shown that the cells in the endothelium will malfunction when exposed to high blood pressure, high levels of cholesterol or insulin (such as the insulin levels found in the most common form of diabetes), smoking, and chronic stress. Under the influence of one or more of these factors, the endothelial cells release harmful chemicals that create a sticky surface. This stickiness attracts other cells that accelerate a multistep process leading to atherosclerosis. This process involves several different types of cells in the vessel wall, and takes many years to develop.

While people often think of atherosclerotic plaque as a mineral-like deposit, it is actually a form of living tissue. Plaque needs blood to support its cells, just as any tissue does. This blood is provided by a series of tiny blood vessels that extend themselves from the original arterial wall into the new growth. However, because of the makeshift nature of these new blood vessels, portions of the plaque sometimes do not receive enough blood. The high concentrations of fat and cholesterol within the plaque also get in the way of supplying the necessary blood and nutrients. When this happens, the inner portion of the plaque dies and is replaced by actual bone tissue in a process called *coronary calcification*. An ultrasound image of an atherosclerotic artery will show these calcified plaques circling around the artery. When doctors cut into an artery at this point, they can actually hear a click as the scalpel breaks the calcified plaques in the wall.

Sometimes a plaque grows so swiftly that the blood vessels are unable to form quickly enough to supply the plaque's cells with oxygen and nutrients. This leads to the development of dead, or necrotic, material.

As the plaque continues to grow, it presses against the cap that covers it. Frequently, plaques sprout small leaks. Blood-clotting factors in the blood then come to the rescue, sealing off these breaks. These repair jobs probably occur at least once per month. It is part of the body's survival system. They temporarily keep necrotic material from escaping into the artery's main channel.

Unfortunately, this solution is often only temporary. The sealant laid down by the blood-clotting factors is converted into additional plaque material over time, which increases the size of the original plaque. This, in turn, increases the amount of obstruction within the artery and makes it more difficult for adequate amounts of blood to reach the heart muscle. However, a blockage by itself is usually not the cause of a heart attack.

A heart attack usually starts when a plaque blocking only 30 to 40 percent of the blood flow ruptures, and the interior escapes. The fatty substances in this decayed material combine with clotting factors in the blood to form a dangerous clot. The fats also trigger inflammation in the blood vessel. This clot may remain at the point of rupture or it may travel down an artery until it hits another plaque or area of obstruction. It then lodges in its new location, often blocking more than 70 percent and sometimes as much as 95 percent of the blood flow. There may even be a complete blockage of the artery. In recent years, doctors have been giving a medication that helps to dissolve this clot in the hours after a heart attack, often with good results.

Only 10 to 20 percent of the plaques in our bodies have a high probability of rupturing. While these rupture-prone plaques usually only obstruct 30 to 40 percent of the vessel opening, they are dangerous because they are inherently unstable. Such plaques account for 80 to 90 percent of all serious heart problems, including heart attacks and chest pain due to inadequate blood flow (also called angina).

Although cholesterol levels in the bloodstream can be reduced in a matter of days or weeks, the effects of lower cholesterol levels on vessel-wall function may require up to six months. Pictures of blood vessels show only small changes in diameter when cholesterol levels are lowered. However, this underestimates the significant changes occurring within plaques as cholesterol levels drop. Changes in the biology of the plaque may help to explain the stabilization of atherosclerotic lesions and the reduction in mortality seen when cholesterol levels are lowered. Both cholesterol levels and the diameter of the blood vessels are simply markers of what is happening inside the plaque itself. It is extremely important to recognize that the coronary vessels are not stiff pipes—the traditional plumber's view of coronary vessels. Rather, they are moving, undulating pipes. Blood-vessel biology is much more complex than the public has been led to believe in the past thirty years.

The blood itself can also promote the process of atherosclerosis by thickening. Increases in blood thickness, or *viscosity*, and elevated levels of a clotting protein called fibrinogen have been reported in patients with high cholesterol levels. The use of cholesterol-lowering drugs has been associated with reductions in both blood viscosity and fibrinogen levels.

Clot formation explains why the most common time for a heart attack is 9 a.m. For unknown reasons, the platelets in the blood are most likely to clot at this time. Various factors decrease the stickiness of these platelets. Aspirin, a drug derived from the willow tree, reduces this stickiness, as do many other natural substances found in the plant world. As we discover more natural medicines, there may be natural alternatives to the common practice of taking aspirin to thin the blood.

The natural remedies for a healthy heart concentrate on improving endothelial cell function. This improved function creates a healthier heart by widening the blood vessels and reducing the chance that a sudden blockage will occur should a plaque burst.

The heart is an extraordinary organ, but it cannot be expected to adapt to overwhelming amounts of damage. Heart disease is both nature and nurture. It is related to your genes, and to your diet and lifestyle. The specific risk factors associated with heart disease are not etched in stone. Just because you have a family history of heart disease, you should not feel that you are doomed to develop heart disease yourself. In the last few years, we have found that it is possible to reverse some of the negative changes in the hearts of patients with heart disease. This means that the amount of vessel blockage in the heart can actually be reduced after a period of diet, exercise, and lifestyle changes. So there really is hope for a reversal of atherosclerosis! In the next chapter, we will look at some of these risk factors, and at rates of heart disease worldwide.

CHAPTER 3

Lessons From Around
the World—
Risk Factors for Heart Disease

Why is heart disease so common in the United States? Heart disease is the number-one killer in this country, yet it kills very few people in some other nations. An American dies of cardiovascular disease every 33 seconds. That is more than 954,000 deaths per year, or more than 42 percent of all deaths each year. The cost of heart disease is estimated by the American Heart Association to be $151.3 billion per year. What is it about our society that makes heart disease so common?

As we look around the world, the rates of heart disease vary widely, as do cholesterol levels. A study was done in 1977 using data collected by the World Health Organization (see Figure 3.1). This international study examined the death rates from coronary heart disease in men thirty-five to seventy-four years of age. There was a big difference in the rates of mortality from this disease. Three countries—Finland, Northern Ireland, and Scotland—had mortality rates of at least 900 persons per 100,000 population. On the other end of the spectrum, Japan had a rate of only 100 per 100,000. That's a ninefold variation in the number of men who died! France, Yugoslavia, and Romania were in the second lowest group among the twenty-seven nations studied, with rates in the 200 to 225 range.

The United States came in with a not-so-spectacular rate of 680 deaths per 100,000, about equal to those of England and Australia. That put Americans in the unenviable position of being in eighth place. Since 1977, there has been a 30 percent drop in the heart disease rate among middle-aged men in the United States, with similar declines for most other population groups. Other nations have not made as much progress in the last twenty years. In fact, as we have spread our Western cultural patterns globally, including our diet and lifestyle habits, we have created an emerging epidemic of chronic disease even within underdeveloped countries that have traditionally had little heart disease. It's important to see why heart disease is so prevalent in the United States.

HEART DISEASE STUDIES
IN THE UNITED STATES

There have been two major studies that looked at the correlation between heart disease and various risk factors in Americans: the Multiple Risk Factor Intervention Trial (MRFIT) and the Framingham study. The first of these studies found a dramatic connection between blood levels of cholesterol and the risk of heart disease. As you can see in Figure 3.2, there is an increase in risk even for people with cholesterol levels in the "normal" range of 180 to 240. There is an even greater jump in risk when the total cholesterol is over 240.

It is tempting to think that this curve explains why so many Americans have heart disease. After all, the average blood level of cholesterol in the 1970s was about 250, and that has dropped to 210 along with about a

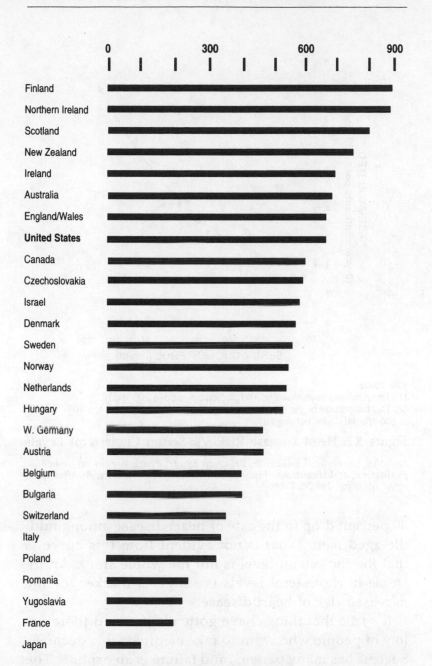

Figure 3.1. Death Rates per 100,000 Population, 1977

Adapted from the Report of the Intersociety Commission for Heart Disease Resources: Optimal resources for the primary prevention of atherosclerotic diseases. *Circulation* 70:1A–205A, 1984.

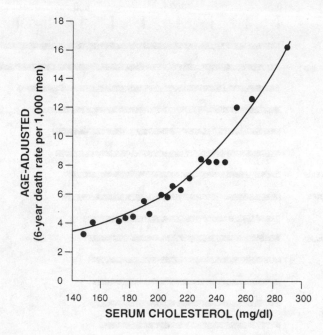

Key points:
(1) The risk increases steadily, and particularly above 200 mg/dL.
(2) The magnitude of the increased risk is large—fourfold in the top 10% as
    compared to the bottom 10%.

Figure 3.2. Heart Disease Risk Vs. Serum Cholesterol Levels

National Cholesterol Education Program Expert Panel. Report on detection,
evaluation, and treatment of high blood cholesterol in adults. *Archives of Internal Medicine* 148:36, 1988.

30 percent drop in the rate of heart disease among middle-aged men. What is not evident from this curve is
that the cholesterol level is not the whole story. An increase in cholesterol levels is simply a marker for the
increased risk of heart disease.

It's true that things have gotten better, and there are
lots of people who want to take credit for this decrease.
Success has many parents, and failure is an orphan. The
parents in this case range from those who perform heart
surgery and operate paramedic services to those who
manufacture cholesterol-lowering drugs.

It is my belief that lifestyle changes have played a large part in the decreases in both cholesterol levels and heart disease rates. These changes include less smoking, better eating habits, and better maintenance of body weight in high-risk individuals. I also believe that we have a long way to go towards reducing heart disease death rates in this country. This is not to say that cholesterol levels are unimportant, but simply to emphasize that there is much more to this story. In order to understand why blood cholesterol level is so important, you have to learn how cholesterol levels are affected by genes, diet, stress, and exercise (factors that will be discussed in Chapters 4 through 7).

Much that we have learned about the causes of heart disease have come from the long-term study conducted in the now-famous town of Framingham, Massachusetts. This study is based on annual medical examinations of people who live there. The original report from the Framingham study, published in 1961, identified serum cholesterol and blood pressure as the two most important risk factors for heart disease after age and sex. Since that original report, there have been almost forty reports extending the initial observations. Some of these reports showed that obesity is another independent risk factor. Others established the roles of total cholesterol, HDL cholesterol, and triglycerides in the development of heart disease. (For more information on these terms, see Chapter 4.)

As in the case of the MRFIT, the Framingham study has shown a strong correlation between total serum cholesterol and coronary heart disease. The Framingham study has also looked at the interaction between cholesterol and other risk factors, including blood pressure, impaired usage within the body of a sugar called glucose (which is also correlated with diabetes), and cigarette smoking. As each of these risk factors is added, the probability of heart disease increases. If your cholesterol level is 335, you would have about *five times* the risk of heart disease as that of someone with a cholesterol count of 195 and high blood pressure. If you have problems suggesting early diabetes, you increase your risk by an additional 50 percent compared with someone who has high blood pressure and high cholesterol. If you add cigarette smoking, there is an additional increase. Table 3.1 shows how these factors add up.

Table 3.1. Eight-Year Probability of Heart Disease Per 1,000 People in Framingham

Risk Factor	Risk
No Risk Factors	less than 10
High Blood Pressure	48
Increase Cholesterol from 195 to 335	210
Add Problems with Glucose	326
Add Cigarette Smoking	459

The key to understanding these risk factors is to realize that they work together in both a positive and negative sense. When you get rid of more than one factor, they work together to give you an even greater reduction in your risk. So if you can reduce several factors at once, you get a bonus by greatly reducing your risk of heart disease. Blood pressure will respond in many cases to a weight loss of as little as 5 to 10 percent of body weight. Cigarette smoking can be stopped. Modest problems with glucose respond to diet, although blood cholesterol levels may not respond to diet as easily.

Remember, you can never be too healthy. The Framingham risk factors are just an easy model to work from. Other factors were not measured in that study. For example, since most people in Framingham eat roughly the same diet, the large international variations in heart disease due to diet are not seen in that study. Other factors that were not measured include changes due to reduced stress and increased levels of physical activity. Your goal should be to go beyond reducing these risk factors. You should aim for optimum health, not just to reduce your risk of heart disease, but also to improve your quality of life and lower your risk of other diseases as well. Look at this challenge in a positive way. You want to reduce your risk in ways that you enjoy. Then you will not only add more years to your life, but more life to your years. Let's take a look at each of these risk factors.

THINGS YOU CAN CHANGE

Obviously, you can't change all of your heart disease risk factors. Your age is a given. So is a family history of heart disease. However, a number of factors are under your control. Let's look at some of them.

Diet

The idea that diet might play a role in atherosclerosis began when cholesterol was found to be part of the plaque in hardened arteries. (For an overall description of how atherosclerosis occurs, see Chapter 2.) About 1910, Russian scientist Nikolai Anitschkow raised the idea that since cholesterol is in the diet, dietary cholesterol caused heart disease. Some studies in humans have shown only minor changes in serum cholesterol when dietary cholesterol intake is increased from 200 to 800 milligrams a day (mg/day). However, the American Heart Association and others recommend consuming less than 300 mg/day. This is not a bad idea, since most sources of dietary cholesterol are also high in fat, which can lead to excess body weight.

The connection between dietary cholesterol and heart disease has since been broadened to include dietary fat. This happened after it was observed that deaths from heart disease in Norway decreased in 1944 and 1945, when the Nazis diverted supplies of dairy fat away from the civilian population. Then in the 1950s, Harvard researchers showed that when you keep dietary fat and calories constant, you can affect serum cholesterol levels by consuming different types of fat. The Harvard researchers found that the saturated fats (fats that are solid at room temperature) found in animals and dairy products raise blood cholesterol levels. On the other hand, the polyunsaturated fats (fats that are very fluid at room temperature) found in vegetable oils such as corn oil, soybean oil, and safflower oil can actually lower cholesterol. The monounsaturated fats (fats that are fluid at room temperature, but less so than polyunsaturated fats) found in nuts, olives, and avocados either do not change cholesterol levels or help to reduce the rise in cholesterol seen in diets with significant amounts of refined sugar. The hydrogenated, or chemically altered, polyunsaturated fats found in many processed foods (also called trans-fatty acids) act more like saturated fats. Fish oils and other similar fats lower the levels of fat in the blood.

Another important factor in the diet is fiber. Fiber, mainly the water-soluble type found in oat bran and some other foods, lowers cholesterol levels by trapping cholesterol-containing particles in the intestine. They are then excreted instead of being assimilated into the body. The body responds by trying to make more cholesterol to replace what was lost. Despite that, there is still a 10 percent reduction in blood cholesterol levels with the use of natural fibers or fiberlike lipid-lowering drugs. (For more information on fiber and fiberlike drugs, see Chapters 10 and 8, respectively.)

To sum up, your diet can affect your cholesterol level in three ways:

- By lowering your body weight
- By reducing your body's cholesterol production
- By increasing the amounts of triglycerides and cholesterol removed from your body

See Chapter 5 for more information on diet.

Physical Activity and Exercise

Even small amounts of physical activity can reduce your risk of heart disease when compared with that of people who are totally sedentary. A shocking 24 percent of all Americans are totally inactive, meaning that whenever they get the urge to exercise, they wait until it passes. Another benefit of exercise is that if you build muscle tissue it changes your body's metabolism for the better by causing you to burn off more fat and sugar for energy. This reduces your blood pressure and the levels of sugar and fats in the blood. See Chapter 7 for guidelines on exercise.

Cigarette Smoking

Cigarette smoking is clearly linked to heart disease. It does increase the risk of lung cancer more than it does the risk of heart disease. However, the net effect of the smoking-heart disease link on the population as a whole is greater because heart disease is more common. The evidence is clear: you should stop smoking. Studies show that you can reduce your risk of heart disease within two years after quitting. Since many people smoke to reduce stress, I've included information on how to stop smoking in Chapter 6, which deals with stress.

Alcohol Use

There is a complex relationship between alcohol use and heart disease. You can slightly reduce your chances of developing heart disease by drinking one to two glasses of beer or wine per day. However, drinking more than two glasses per day increases your blood pressure and your chances of developing other chronic diseases. If you can drink alcohol in moderation, then you can continue to have one or two drinks per day. This probably acts as a stress reducer. On the other hand, the tremendous social and medical costs of alcoholism make it wrong for me to recommend alcohol to anyone who is not already drinking. It is particularly important that anyone with a family history of alcoholism avoid alcohol entirely. See Chapter 6 for more information.

Stress

While it is difficult to document the effects of stress on heart disease, it is clear that constant stress has a very negative effect. Research results are very sketchy concerning possible connections between heart disease and any particular personality type. The so-called Type A personality, characterized as hard-driving and ambitious, can also be present in a totally healthy individual who uses that personality to develop a healthful, structured personal exercise and diet program. Instead, many researchers consider unexpressed internalized anger to be a factor in heart disease. Reducing your overall stress level also increases your quality of life. I discuss stress reduction at length in Chapter 6.

Obesity

Obesity is a risk factor for heart disease, even if your cholesterol levels are normal. It increases your risk by promoting high blood pressure and high levels of fats and sugar in the blood. What's more, the wall of the heart must grow to be able to pump the additional blood volume required in obese individuals at their higher blood pressures. This can make the heart less efficient. The diet recommendations in this book will not only help to lower cholesterol levels but help you achieve and maintain a healthy body weight as well. There is a simple seven-step diet plan in Chapter 5 that will start you on your way to eliminating this important risk factor.

High Blood Pressure

With the possible exception of high cholesterol levels, high blood pressure is the most consistent risk factor for heart disease. High blood pressure reflects the influences of stress and body weight. A 5 to 10 percent loss in body weight can normalize blood pressure in many individuals. The lower the blood pressure, the better, even within the so-called normal range. Blood pressure is measured with two numbers called the systolic and diastolic pressures. The systolic is the highest pressure your heart pumps against and the diastolic is the lowest. An average healthy blood pressure is 120/80 (systolic/diastolic). High blood pressure begins at 150/90. Just as with cholesterol, you can improve your health even when your current blood pressure is below the level at which doctors would say you have high blood pressure. When you exercise, one of the benefits is a further lowering of blood pressure even if your pressure is in what is considered to be the normal range. Remember, you can never get too healthy when it comes to blood pressure. The better the tone of your blood vessels and the lower your blood pressure, the less work your heart has to do in pumping blood around your body. See Chapter 7 for more information on exercise.

Blood Clotting Factors

I know this sounds like a factor you can't control, but diet and the use of natural remedies can affect this process. Various components of the same blood-clotting mechanism that insures you don't bleed to death from a paper cut can also increase your risk of heart disease. This is especially true when levels of certain forms of one of these clotting proteins, fibrinogen, are elevated. One of the ways that fish oil helps protect your heart is by decreasing the stickiness of the platelet cells that help to form blood clots. Aspirin, a natural product from the willow tree, also works in this way. For more information on natural therapies, see Chapter 10.

The international data on the rates of heart disease show that diet and lifestyle are clearly important in determining whether a genetic tendency for heart disease will actually result in heart disease. However, not everyone who fails to follow a healthy lifestyle develops heart disease. Some people are extremely lucky. Eubie Blake, the jazz musician, lived to be 104 years old despite smoking and drinking every day of his adult life. He commented, "If I'd have known I was going to live this long, I would've taken better care of myself!" Unfortunately, not all of us are blessed with such good genes.

Cholesterol levels are not genetically determined. Genetics is important, but the diet, exercise patterns, and lifestyle of the individual are closely related to the incidence of heart disease and many other diseases. As you will see in Chapter 4, the cholesterol in your diet does not always turn into cholesterol in the bloodstream. Other factors may be more important, such as the food's fat content and the total calorie intake measured against your level of physical activity. There are also natural products that can lower your risk of heart disease in many different ways. In order to fully appreciate the alternatives available, I will now show you how cholesterol levels are controlled and how they lead to atherosclerosis.

CHAPTER 4

The Cholesterol Thermostat

Scientists have learned about cholesterol in fits and starts. There would be a major break-through, and then years or even decades would pass before the next big discovery. It has now been over 150 years since the first research was done on cholesterol. During that time, researchers have isolated it, determined its precise chemical structure, and discovered the many functions it performs.

We have learned that cholesterol is so essential to life that it is used in every single cell of the human body. Scientists have also determined that some people are genetically predisposed to a high cholesterol level, although diet and lifestyle changes can help almost everyone lower their cholesterol naturally. The basis for this genetic predisposition is an alteration in what I call the cholesterol thermostat. Let's look at what cholesterol is and how it goes astray, leading to atherosclerosis.

THE SCIENCE OF CHOLESTEROL

In 1815, a French chemist, Michel Chevreul, identified

cholesterol as a white, flaky substance different from other waxy substances. In 1824, he found that cholesterol is produced by the liver and is found in bile, which helps to digest fatty foods in the intestine. Chevreul was the first person to give cholesterol a name: cholesterine. The modern name, cholesterol, is actually a combination of the Greek words *chole*, meaning bile, and *stereos*, meaning solid. Cholesterol was later found in human blood and brain tissue, as well as in chicken eggs. Even more importantly, cholesterol was discovered in arteries that had plaque buildup.

In 1856, a German pathologist named Rudolf Virchow began studying what we know today as atherosclerosis, or hardening of the arteries. He found that significant changes occur within the arterial walls during the process of plaque buildup. The actual hardening, he discovered, was due to the formation of bone tissue in the artery wall. Thus, the word "atherosclerosis" comes from the Greek words for gruel (*athero*) and hardening (*sclerois*). In the early twentieth century, scientists learned how fats and cholesterol work their way into the artery wall to produce the dreaded buildup of plaque. In 1910, German researcher Adolf Windaus and two colleagues found that there is a much higher concentration of cholesterol in an aorta (the body's main artery) damaged by atherosclerosis than there is in normal tissue. Later, Nikolai Anitschkow fed cholesterol to healthy rabbits and was able to produce a fatty buildup similar to that seen in early atherosclerosis.

Slowly but surely, the connections among cholesterol, atherosclerosis, and diet are being discovered. At the UCLA laboratories of Dr. Linda Demer and Dr. Alan Fogelman, scientists are focusing on atherosclerosis at the cellular level, and on the role of bone formation in this process. They have discovered the biological basis for some of Virchow's original observations by using cutting-edge methods of molecular and cellular biology.

CONTROLLING THE CREATION OF CHOLESTEROL: THE CHOLESTEROL THERMOSTAT

Obviously, the main role of cholesterol in the body is not the production of heart disease. We now know that cholesterol is produced by the liver and other tissues for several vital purposes. We'll look at how cholesterol is normally used in the body, and at the triglycerides, the fats associated with cholesterol. We'll then see how cholesterol and triglycerides are delivered throughout the body, and how this transport system can break down, contributing to the development of atherosclerosis.

Cholesterol's Function Within the Body

Cholesterol serves various important functions. It is a vital component of the microscopic wall, or membrane, that surrounds each cell, providing the cell with support and protection. Cholesterol is required for the formation of vitamin D, and of the hormones testosterone, estrogen, progesterone, and cortisol. In the brain and spinal cord, cholesterol serves as part of the insulation that covers your nerve cells and keeps your nerve signals going to the right locations. Cholesterol also plays a key role in the formation of bile. Without cholesterol, your body would be unable to digest the fats found in many of the foods you eat.

Scientists have discovered that most of the cholesterol in the human body is produced by its own cells, particularly the cells of the liver. They have found that cholesterol formation is controlled much as the thermostat in your home controls temperature. When the cholesterol level in the blood rises because of diet, the production of cholesterol by the liver decreases in an attempt to keep the level of cholesterol in the blood constant. Just like the thermostat in your house, the system works to maintain a certain blood level of cholesterol. This feedback loop is known as *homeostasis*.

The problem for many of us is that the thermostat was set thousands of years ago, when cholesterol, fat, and calories were deficient in our diets. In the modern diet, that is simply not the case. It would be similar to having your thermostat set in Rochester, New York, even though your house was located in Tucson, Arizona. Cholesterol levels rise because the thermostat was set in a different environment.

Dr. Marvin Siperstein, now at the University of California, San Francisco, made an important but underappreciated discovery a while back. He was studying cholesterol control in the livers of different animal species. He found that every species he studied controls its cholesterol production in the liver except for the trout. What made the trout different?

Dr. Siperstein couldn't understand the problem until he visited the fish hatchery. There, he learned that all the trout he had studied had liver tumors. Thus, their cholesterol production was uncontrolled. This led to the discovery that runaway cholesterol production occurs in tumor cells, while normal tissues have finely tuned cholesterol thermostats. Cholesterol is so essential to cell function that liver cancer cells can be killed by cutting off their ability to make cholesterol. (Recently, Japanese scientists have tested cholesterol-lowering drugs in the treatment of liver cancer with encouraging results. Other scientists are studying limonene and geraniol, substances derived from citrus-fruit peels, to see if these chemicals can inhibit cholesterol creation in cancer cells.)

Cholesterol comes from two main sources: your diet (*exogenous cholesterol*) and the cholesterol your body manufactures on its own (*endogenous cholesterol*). I'll refer to them as "outside cholesterol" and "inside cholesterol," respectively.

The vast majority of the cholesterol circulating in your blood is inside cholesterol. If you ate a diet that was very low in cholesterol and fat, your body would be able to use the small amounts of cholesterol and fat (triglycerides) in your diet effectively. Under those conditions, which prevailed 10,000 years ago, dietary fat and cholesterol would be an important supplement to your body's own production. However, in our modern state of fat-and-calorie overload, we get far more of these substances than our bodies can possibly use. Even worse, the high calorie and fat content in today's typical diets can stimulate excess cholesterol production, making it harder for cholesterol to be removed from the bloodstream.

Outside cholesterol enters the bloodstream from the intestines. The intestinal walls absorb the cholesterol from the partially digested food and package it, along with several other substances, into special carrier molecules called *chylomicrons*. Chylomicrons begin to enter your bloodstream within minutes after you eat a meal containing fat. Since fatty foods take a long time to be fully digested, these chylomicrons continue to enter the bloodstream for several hours after you finish eating. Once they are in your blood, they travel throughout your blood vessels. In time, they pass through the liver and are processed much like the cholesterol packages that your body makes on its own.

Cholesterol's Transport Partner: The Triglycerides

Cholesterol does not travel around the bloodstream by itself. It is generally packaged with fats called *triglycerides*. Triglycerides are the body's preferred form of energy storage. The only reason you can survive without food for extended periods is because of your triglyceride stores. These triglycerides make up about 95 percent of the fat in the foods you eat, and the vast majority of the fat in your body. Your liver can also convert carbohydrates into triglycerides for storage.

Triglycerides are constructed from substances known as fatty acids. When a triglyceride is needed for energy, it is broken down within the fat cell into three fatty acids—the "tri" in "triglyceride." It is then transported to the site in the body where the energy is needed, such as the legs if you are walking.

Your body can make some fatty acids. However, there are two fatty acids that must be obtained from the diet: linolenic and linoleic acid. These are called *essential fatty acids*. So you do need to eat a small amount of dietary fat each day, about 5 to 10 percent of your total calories. Theoretically, you could have a fatty-acid deficiency. In all my years of clinical practice, though, I have never lost a patient to this deficiency. On the contrary, excess consumption of fats of all types is a much more frequent problem.

Cholesterol Packaged for Transport: The Three Types of Cholesterol

Earlier in this century, researchers began looking at the different *lipoproteins*—the fat-and-protein packages that travel through the bloodstream—to see what roles these substances might play in the development of coronary artery disease. This has led to our current understanding about "good" and "bad" cholesterol. At the same time, several large studies examined the long-term health consequences of different levels of cholesterol in the blood. These studies confirmed that excess cholesterol in the bloodstream can cause major damage to your cardiovascular system, resulting in various forms of heart disease and even death.

So what makes good cholesterol good and bad cholesterol bad? As I noted earlier, all of your cells need cholesterol, yet they have only a limited ability to produce it. In order to get cholesterol where it is needed, the liver has developed a complex system that bundles cholesterol and triglycerides together into lipoproteins. We can think of the lipoproteins as delivery trucks, with the liver serving as the truck depot. These lipoprotein trucks have specially designed loading ramps made up of proteins, called *apolipoproteins*. These ramps fit into specially designed docking bays called *receptors* on the cells of various organs, such as the liver and muscles.

Each loading ramp also contains an onboard computer that tells the delivery truck where the cargo of cholesterol and triglycerides is headed. It might be going to the muscles to be burned, to the fat tissues to be stored, or back to the liver to be converted into bile acids or hormones.

The amount of cholesterol produced by the liver is controlled by signals from the liver cells, which stimulate the activity of an enzyme known as *HMG-CoA reductase*. (An enzyme is a special protein that carries out chemical reactions.) This enzyme is critical in the production of cholesterol. We can think of it as being the chief dispatcher that determines how many lipoprotein trucks will go out on their routes each day.

There are three lipoproteins in your bloodstream: very-low-density lipoprotein (*VLDL*), low-density lipoprotein (*LDL*), and high-density lipoprotein (*HDL*). Two of these (VLDL and HDL) are produced by your liver, while LDL is created in the bloodstream from VLDL under certain circumstances. These lipoprotein trucks carry a variety of cargo, which changes as each truck moves along its route in the bloodstream. Let's look at each type of lipoprotein separately.

The VLDL truck carries several types of cargo as it leaves the liver depot. It has relatively little protein and cholesterol in its shipment, but carries a lot of triglycerides. Because of these characteristics, VLDLs are the largest and least soluble lipoprotein trucks. They are the least stable, too. The VLDL truck also carries several different kinds of loading ramps.

When the VLDL truck arrives at a particular tissue, it encounters an enzyme called *lipoprotein lipase* in the tiny blood vessels on the surface. This enzyme sets the cargo-unloading process in motion. The first thing that the lipoprotein lipase does is to hook up with loading ramp apolipoprotein C, or *Apo C*. Lipoprotein lipase then unloads some of the triglycerides, which are then used for energy or stored as body fat.

As the VLDL continues on its route, it gradually releases its triglycerides. When it has lost most of its triglycerides, it is called a *VLDL remnant*, a big, half-empty truck. Eventually, all of the triglyceride cargo is unloaded and the VLDL becomes triglyceride-poor. Yet because the VLDL did not unload its cholesterol cargo at the same time, the end result is a lipoprotein truck that still carries a relatively rich load of cholesterol. It also still has its apolipoprotein B, or *Apo B*, loading ramp. This lipoprotein is now an LDL truck. Most of the cholesterol in the bloodstream is found in the LDL trucks. The remaining cholesterol cargo is carried on the VLDL and the HDL trucks. (To learn how your doctor figures how much of each lipoprotein is in your blood, see "Doing the Cholesterol Math.")

Not Enough Docking Bays: LDL Cholesterol Goes Astray

The cholesterol in the various lipoprotein trucks is used for the essential functions I mentioned earlier: hormone

---

Doing the Cholesterol Math

Your doctor may send you for blood tests to indicate your levels of triglycerides and the various forms of cholesterol. When you get the results of your cholesterol test from your doctor, he or she is using a formula that approximates the amounts of LDL cholesterol and HDL cholesterol, as well as the cholesterol carried on VLDL. It works like this:

Total Cholesterol = LDL Cholesterol + Triglycerides divided by 5 + HDL Cholesterol

The triglycerides must be divided by 5 because VLDLs, the main carriers of triglycerides, are 20 percent cholesterol. The HDL cholesterol is measured by a special method that takes advantage of the size differential between the smaller HDL particles and the other particles. It is important that this test be done while you are fasting. While the total cholesterol does not change after a meal, the triglyceride level often does.

---

production, nerve insulation, cell wall creation, and so forth. When a cell needs cholesterol, a receptor docking bay on the cell's membrane routes an LDL truck out of the bloodstream. At this point, the Apo B loading ramp helps bind the LDL to the receptor. About 80 percent of these LDL receptor docking bays are found in the liver, while the remaining 20 percent are found in the other tissues.

The work of these receptors is crucial to your health. Even though the body has an ability to produce new receptors and eliminate them when they are not needed, its flexibility is limited. When your receptors are in proper working order and you have enough of them to pull all of your LDL into the body's cells, you should not have a problem with high cholesterol levels. There will be an equilibrium between the supply of receptors and the demands that you place on them.

However, a problem arises if your body's cholesterol thermostat causes it to produce too much cholesterol on its own or if you eat too much of the wrong foods. If that happens, too many LDL trucks will arrive at the receptor docking bays, and many of the trucks will not be captured. Such runaway trucks will simply keep on driving around your bloodstream until the drivers decide to pull over. Unfortunately, this is often in the wall of an artery.

Did you ever wonder how cholesterol is trapped in the artery wall? It actually passes through the wall's surface quite easily, since the membrane covering the inner surface of the artery is made of fat. Once the LDL truck lodges in the artery wall, it becomes trapped in a three-dimensional cagework of fibers. These fibers are secreted by the cells of the vessel wall into the space just underneath the membrane that covers the inside vessel wall.

Once the trucks are trapped, they become *oxidized*. Oxidation is the chemical change that occurs when certain substances are exposed to oxygen. Two common examples are the rusting of a car exposed to the elements and the process that turns the cut surface of an apple from white to brown. In the case of our LDL trucks, you can think of them as being full of butter. The butter is now going rancid and the trucks are rusting. The cells of the artery wall shed chemical wastes that can cause oxidation of the trapped LDL.

Does the butter on the LDL trucks have to go rancid? No. Substances known as *antioxidants* serve as preservatives and keep the butter from spoiling. If antioxidants are carried on the LDL truck itself, or if they are present in the area where they are trapped, they can prevent this oxidation from occurring.

Vitamin E, a fat-soluble antioxidant, is one of the most effective in preventing this oxidation. There are many other natural antioxidants as well. Iron, on the other hand, stimulates the oxidation of LDL. Studies from Scandinavia show that a high level of iron in the blood may be related to atherosclerosis in some people.

Once it goes rancid, the LDL attracts other cells into the space it occupies in the artery wall. These cells eat the rancid LDL and become *foam cells*. Foam cells fill up with cholesterol and ultimately burst open when they die. In the process, various factors stimulate the growth of smooth muscle cells in the artery wall, which means that there is an overgrowth of muscle. Over a number of years, all of these cellular events contribute to the progress of atherosclerosis.

Tow Trucks to the Rescue: The Good HDL

It's easy to see why LDL is called the bad cholesterol. It is responsible for the formation of plaque in arterial walls. This can lead to atherosclerosis and other debilitating conditions. But what about the good cholesterol?

HDL is the truck that helps carry cholesterol back to the liver. HDL is produced principally by the liver and intestines, although some other tissues can also manufacture it to a limited degree. Compared with the other lipoproteins, HDL carries very little fat. It also has a cargo that is only 20 percent cholesterol, which is much less than the LDL and VLDL trucks. Because of these characteristics, HDL is the most soluble and easily transported of the three lipoprotein trucks.

HDL is known as the good cholesterol for good reason. Working with its apolipoprotein E, or *Apo E*, loading ramp, which in this case acts like a towing mechanism, HDL is able to tow the VLDL remnants in the blood back to the liver before they can be converted into LDL. HDL can also inhibit the LDL oxidation process by releasing a chemical that keeps the butter on the LDL trucks from going rancid. Once in the liver, the VLDL remnants are broken down into their basic components. Some of the cholesterol in the remnant is converted to bile acids and excreted into the intestinal tract for removal from the body. The remaining portion is used to construct a new VLDL truck so the entire cycle can begin again.

THE REASONS PEOPLE DEVELOP ATHEROSCLEROSIS—AND WAYS TO STOP IT

It should be noted that some people are genetically predisposed to high LDL levels. For these people, dietary restraint is not enough. These individuals have inherited a genetic defect that makes it more difficult for them to process the LDL in their blood. They may have received a defective gene for the LDL receptor from one or both parents, so their bodies cannot create enough docking bays. One in a million individuals has two of these bad genes. A person with this problem usually dies of heart disease in his or her twenties or thirties. A liver transplant, which gives the recipient normal receptors, is the only answer.

One in 500 people has one defective gene and one normal gene. People with this problem have cholesterol levels that can range from 300 to 500 milligrams a deciliter (mg/dL), compared with a normal, safe cholesterol level of 200 mg/dL or less. The excess LDL makes its way to the arterial walls. By the time these people are in their forties and fifties, they often have advanced atherosclerosis.

The majority of people who go on to develop heart disease have none of these rare LDL defects, but have what is called *mixed hyperlipidemia*. This is characterized by a rise in both cholesterol and triglyceride levels, and is often accompanied by obesity, diabetes, and a high-fat diet.

On the other hand, there is a clear correlation between high HDL levels and a low incidence of atherosclerosis and other cardiovascular diseases. In fact, the level of HDL cholesterol is the best predictor of future coronary difficulties in people over fifty years of age. This makes HDL level an even better heart disease predictor than total cholesterol and LDL levels. Moreover, even when total cholesterol levels are greater than they should be, a high ratio of HDL to LDL lipoproteins seems to have a protective effect. One study found that the risk of coronary heart disease declines by 2 to 3 percent for every 1 mg/dL rise in the HDL level.

These discoveries suggest that a multipronged, natural approach to your battle against cholesterol will be the most effective. You should reduce your overall fat and calorie consumption to minimize the amount of LDL circulating in your bloodstream. However, you should also take positive steps to increase your HDL level independently of your total cholesterol count. Losing weight can lead to a decrease in triglycerides and an increase in HDL cholesterol. Giving up smoking has a number of benefits, including a reduction in LDL oxidation. Using antioxidants such as vitamin E can help prevent oxidation of LDL as well. Finally, exercising can increase HDL and lower total cholesterol. A number of natural products also have antioxidants that act like vitamin E to counteract the pro-oxidants in our foods and the environment.

These different strategies work together so that the total is greater than the sum of the parts. 2+2=5! Scientists call such combinations synergistic. In the battle to stop the process of atherosclerosis, multiple approaches work best. There is no single magic bullet. Natural therapies only produce the greatest improvements when used in combination with a healthy diet and exercise. In fact, even the most powerful cholesterol-lowering drugs can be neutralized by poor diets and lifestyles.

As we've seen, heart disease is caused by much more than cholesterol. The level of cholesterol in the blood provides a clue that something is wrong, but nothing more. Atherosclerosis is a long process that starts in childhood and progresses into old age. Usually, heart disease results from a thermostat that is genetically set at too high a level in an individual who is too sedentary and who eats a diet that is too high in fat and cholesterol. Frequently, there is also an elevation in the level of triglycerides. This sets the stage for atherosclerosis and other cardiovascular diseases. Yet even with improved diet and exercise, many patients need additional help in reaching their desired cholesterol level.

Are drugs the answer? Not necessarily. Natural therapies have been discovered that can slow atherosclerosis in the laboratory. These findings are giving us new hope that we can one day reduce or even eliminate heart disease. This may seem like a pipe dream, but only a generation ago clogged arteries were considered an inevitable part of aging. We have come a long way, yet we still have far to go. Fortunately, new breakthroughs in the area of plant extracts and nutritional therapies are giving us new tools in the battle against heart disease.

Your body is an amazing biological machine, but it can only tolerate so much abuse. You need to be on the same team with your body by reducing the amount of fat, calories, and cholesterol you consume. In the next chapter, I'll show you how.

CHAPTER 5

Eat to Your Heart's Content—
The Skinny on
Lowering Cholesterol Levels

Whenever I talk to someone about diet, a grim look crosses their face. The word is scary, implying denial. But in this chapter, instead of deprivation, we are going to talk about eating strategies.

My goal is to change your eating behaviors. Sometimes, my advice won't seem to make sense. For example, what is wrong with fruit-flavored nonfat yogurt? Nutritionally, nothing. However, there is plenty wrong from a behavioral point of view. Fruit-flavored nonfat yogurt tastes like ice cream, and thus can encourage a craving for sweets and fats. It's all in the way you taste your food, and what triggers binge eating for you will not affect someone else. We are all different in how we taste food.

Poor eating behavior leads to problems with obesity. Obesity, medically defined as being overfat, is the most common nutritional disorder in the United States today. The most common causes of obesity are eating too much, frequently in response to stress, and exercising too little. Many of us have invested our foods with great power over our emotions. We eat for entertainment, or to relieve boredom. However, you can take control of your eating and exercise habits, and of your reactions to stress.

I am not going to tell you to never eat something. If you want an ice cream on a hot day, go ahead. Rather, I hope to convince you that you can change your taste buds and enjoy a healthy diet without giving up all of your pleasures in life. I have many patients who watch what they eat most of the time but feel free to splurge occasionally. If you follow my plan, a strange thing will happen. Soon you won't want those same high-fat foods as much. You will like your new shape, and your taste buds will change. (The same thing will happen to a taste for very salty foods.) It has been shown that preventing disease is not as much of a motivator for changing lifestyle as is looking and feeling better. Before we get to my suggestions, let's first look at why our diets are so unhealthy.

THE PERILS OF THE MODERN DIET

The U.S. Department of Agriculture, in an ongoing survey of the nation's health, has found that obesity is on the rise. About 24 percent of the Americans surveyed between 1976 and 1980 were obese. However, about 32 percent of those surveyed between 1988 and 1994 were obese. That is a 30 percent increase. How can this happen at a time when Americans are more health-conscious than ever? Part of it is a hectic lifestyle, with no time to prepare healthy meals or to exercise. However, another important factor is an emphasis on fat content, and a reduced awareness of total calories. Thus, we cut fat but increase portion sizes and consume more sugary snacks, unaware that sugar can be converted to fat.

There are also hidden fats in our foods. They are

there for one good reason: Fat helps sell food. Food is sold on the basis of taste, cost, and convenience. Fat makes food taste better, so it can be used to disguise poor ingredients. Foods made with fat are also easier to process and handle. Actually, when food manufacturers take out the fat, they have to put something back in to enhance the flavor. That something is usually sugar in one of its many forms (maltodextrin, corn sugar, dates, honey, etc.). You end up with the same number of calories or even more. Instead of losing weight, you stay the same or actually gain weight!

Our food supply was not always as high in fat as it is today. For most of humankind's existence on this planet, we have eaten low-fat, high-fiber foods. Today, we go to a steakhouse instead and eat a fourteen-ounce steak with more than 1,200 calories and lots of saturated fat. If your taste buds enjoy fast food, you may go to a fast-food chain and have a big double burger, fries, and a chocolate shake, and wind up consuming 1,300 calories. These are huge numbers of calories for the small amount of nutrients you receive.

French fries are a good example of what's wrong with the modern diet. The making of French fries in this country is carried out with the precision of a space mission. The deep fryers in all the major fast-food chains are carefully programmed within a tenth of a second to carry out a very sophisticated cooking process. The water at the center of the potato boils, depositing the meat of the potato on the outside wall of the French fry just as that wall is browning in the oil. One species of potato, the Russell Burbank, is used for French fries because its low sugar content keeps the French fry from turning black. The oil once had lard in it (the secret ingredient). Then the name was changed to "beef fat." After the public became aware of this ruse, the beef fat was replaced with hydrogenated soybean oil, which at least did not have cholesterol. This new oil has the same high boiling point, so it can still perform its magic on the outside of the French fry.

Is all of this engineering worth it? You bet. French fries bring customers into fast-food chains so they will buy high-profit items such as the colas and other carbonated beverages. Competition and economics have made all this happen. I have used the example of the French fry to indicate the process by which many of our foods have been changed, "perfected," and made to taste better than ever before. Is there another way to make a fry? Yes. You can air-cook sliced potato or dip it in egg white and bake it with some spicy dressing. But compare the air-cooked fry against the deep-fried French fry, and guess which wins the taste test every time: the high-fat fry. No question about it.

DIET AND BEHAVIOR—AND FAT

So is changing the way you eat a hopeless cause? The answer is a resounding *no*! My own research has shown that men and women in this country can be taught to eat reduced-fat and nonfat foods in eight to twelve weeks. They not only learn to like the taste of the food, but after a while their palates change and they don't even enjoy the high-fat foods they used to eat. That's right. Presented with a high-fat snack, these people will get upset stomachs, diarrhea, and gas. This is called *fatty-food intolerance*. When patients tell me about these symptoms, I always reassure them that there is nothing wrong medically, and encourage them to keep up the good work.

It is more important to reduce the fat in your diet than any other single nutrient. (Fiber is an important nonnutrient that I discuss in Chapter 10.) Fat is calorie-rich, with nine calories per gram. However, reducing your fat intake will not necessarily solve your diet problems. If you just substitute refined sugar for fat, you may end up with higher cholesterol levels and no weight loss. Along with reducing fat in the diet, I will teach you how to control your food portions. So this will not be a diet, but a strategy for eating. I want to inspire you to change.

You can get more information from lots of sources. Yet information and education do not change eating behavior. Good eating behavior will be sustained because it makes you feel more energetic, allows you to wear more fashionable clothes, and brings you the admiration of your friends.

While information does not change behavior, you need some information to be able to understand how to use the strategies I am going to show you. You may be surprised to learn that the cholesterol you eat in your diet does not translate directly into increased cholesterol in your bloodstream. As you learned in Chapter 4, your body regulates cholesterol carefully. Most of the cholesterol circulating in your bloodstream is made by your body instead of coming from your food supply. So why is there all this hoopla about cholesterol-free foods? Most high-cholesterol foods such as red meats are also high in fat and carry extra hidden calories. The most important influence on your cholesterol levels is actually the fat and calorie content of your foods rather than their cholesterol content.

Dietary fat and calorie consumption are the most common factors in bringing out a genetic tendency to high cholesterol. The level of genetic predisposition to high cholesterol varies, but these same genes may also cause you to have high blood pressure, diabetes, and even gout. The good news is that if you have these genetic characteristics, you will have the most remarkable responses to diet. In some of my patients, I have seen decreases in cholesterol levels of up to 40 percent from weight loss and a low-fat diet. The decreases are even greater when the patient increases his or her amount of exercise, because the increased muscle mass removes more of the cholesterol and triglycerides from the bloodstream. You can have this type of high-cholesterol problem and be only mildly overweight. A loss of only twenty pounds of extra fat from around the middle (resulting in a one- to two-inch reduction in waist circumference) will significantly reduce your cholesterol levels. For more information on genetics, cholesterol, and fats, see Chapter 4.

Nothing that I have said so far applies to you if you are thin and have high cholesterol. (Increasing your fiber intake can still be important even if you are thin. See Chapter 10.) In this situation, your cholesterol is elevated because your cholesterol thermostat (as discussed in Chapter 4) is set too high. You need something more than diet to reduce your risk of heart disease. I have had patients who were not overweight at all but had high cholesterol levels. Their diets helped to control their cholesterol, but diet alone would not get their cholesterol levels into a healthy range. The strategies for eating I describe in this chapter won't hurt you, but they will have less of an effect on your cholesterol levels than if you have extra body fat. However, you should consider these diet suggestions anyway to maximize the effectiveness of the natural therapies discussed in Chapters 9 and 10.

THE IMPORTANCE OF PROTEIN

Whenever you concentrate on one food component to the exclusion of others, you run the risk of a deficiency. Many people who are trying to eliminate fat and red meat go overboard. They eat less chicken and fish as well, and wind up being protein deficient. This can lead to a loss of muscle mass, which results in higher cholesterol levels. Typically, most diet programs suggest that 20 percent of your total calories should be in the form of protein. Recently, the concept of low-carbohydrate dieting has been revived, in which protein intakes of 30 percent are recommended. Unfortunately, these diets also recommend a fat intake of 30 percent. This will not, in my opinion, lower cholesterol levels unless you exercise enough to burn off the additional fat calories.

I will ask you to maintain a good protein intake. Protein helps to build muscle and will help reduce your appetite between meals. A moderate-protein, moderate-carbohydrate, and low-fat diet is best. Increasing your protein intake will not be harmful as long as your kidneys function normally. In fact, if you exercise you can eat as much as 40 percent of your total calories as protein without any health problems. When combined with weightlifting, this higher level of protein intake may produce more efficient increases in muscle mass than lower protein intakes. So if you want to build muscle, you may wish to use larger protein portions as well as cutting your fat consumption.

There are a number of protein powders on the market that will make it easy for you to get enough protein. Try having a protein drink in the middle of the morning and another drink in the middle of the afternoon. You should also increase the recommended protein portions from three ounces to six ounces at lunch and dinner. (For information on a special type of protein called soy protein, see Chapter 10.) However, if you are eating more protein, you had better be exercising. Otherwise, you will gain fat tissue. Excess calories of any type will lead to body fat. My research group at UCLA is currently experimenting with high-protein, very-low-fat diets in heart disease patients to see if it is practical to build back muscle tissue lost due to inactivity and decreased protein intake. My own experience tells me that this is entirely possible. In Chapter 7, you will learn how to burn off body fat by exercising regularly and building muscle. Increasing your protein intake is one important part of that strategy.

DR. HEBER'S EASY SEVEN-STEP STRATEGY TO REDUCE FAT

While you do need a small amount of fat in your diet to ensure good health, in our society you can virtually get this amount by accident. You can get enough of the essential fatty acids, linoleic and linolenic acid, with a diet that is only 5 to 10 percent fat. With my seven-step strategy, you will simply be minimizing or avoiding foods such as mayonnaise, shortening, salad dressings, and nuts. While there are distinctions in the chemical composition of various types of fats (saturated, unsaturated, etc.), for now just focus on reducing your overall fat consumption, and everything else will fall into place.

I will now describe some proven strategies for eating less fat. My suggestions are simple and easy to remember. My patients remember them when they leave the examination room and are tempted by high-fat desserts. A gradual change is like stretching a rubber band: it can always snap back to its original position. My recommended changes are like breaking a rubber band. My goal is to permanently change your taste buds so you never go back to eating the high-fat foods that are helping keep your body fat and your cholesterol levels too high. This is a well-recognized goal of almost every program that has been devised to reduce cholesterol levels and the risk of heart disease.

Here is the seven-step strategy in compact form (also see Table 5.1). Consider giving up:

- Nuts, including peanuts, macadamia nuts, peanut butter, and pistachios

- Salad dressings made with oil

- Mayonnaise, margarine, and butter

- Red meat, including veal, beef, pork, and lamb

- Fatty fish, including salmon, trout, and catfish

- Cheese and cheese pizza

- Nonfat and low-fat flavored yogurt and ice cream

Let's look at each step in a little more detail.

First, I want you to minimize the intake of *nuts*, including peanuts, macadamia nuts, peanut butter, and pistachios. These are very high in fat. It is true that nuts contain the monounsaturated fatty acids found in olive oil and avocados, but if we are going to cut our fat calories, we have to cut out all types of fat. Instead of nuts, choose a healthy alternative. For example, if you are on a plane, have a beverage instead of the package of peanuts you are offered. Some airlines offer nut-shaped pretzels with half the calories of nuts. At home, have air-popped popcorn. Don't worry about two or three nuts in a salad or pasta dish on occasion, but don't eat a bowlful. That is a good way to gain weight.

Second, consider giving up *salad dressings made with oil*. Switch to wine vinegar, rice vinegar, or balsamic vinegar instead. You could also mix mustard with rice vinegar to make a Dijon-like dressing. Some vinegars now have various spices mixed into them to enhance their flavor. I have even found a raspberry wine vinegar. The key to a delicious fat-free salad is to make the salad out of dark green, leafy lettuce. I often refer to iceberg lettuce as dressing-deficient lettuce, because you have to douse it in dressing to cover up the watery taste of the lettuce. Darker green lettuces are also much better sources of certain nutrients, such as folate. Remember to exclude beans (healthy, but they add calories) and croutons from your salad. Put these suggestions into practice as you go a salad bar and you will wind up with a much healthier meal.

Third, consider giving up *mayonnaise, margarine,* and *butter.* Did you know that fat-free margarine is 100 percent fat? There are five calories per serving and five calories from fat, according to the label. Last time I checked, five divided by five was 100 percent. However, the U.S. Department of Agriculture says that if something has less than 0.5 gram of fat per serving (which is about five calories) it can be called fat-free. The same holds true for fat-free mayonnaise. Substitute fruit jam for margarine in the morning and eat your bread warm so it is moist. You can occasionally use roasted garlic as a butter substitute. I admit the taste is different, but the use of margarine, butter, and mayonnaise is an acquired taste.

Fourth, consider giving up all *red meat.* This includes veal, beef, pork, and lamb. Even when you cut away the visible fat from red meat, there is still plenty of fat between the muscle fibers. A fourteen-ounce piece of prime rib can have more than 1,200 calories and 50 grams of fat. These are all of the calories and fat that an average five-foot-tall woman needs for an entire day and over half the calories needed by an average five-foot, ten-inch man. When the USDA talks about a serving of meat, they are referring to a three-ounce portion—about the size of the palm of your hand. This is something you rarely get in restaurants. Most of my patients say they have already cut down on their red-meat intake. However, I am suggesting that you consider making it a rare part of your diet or even give it up entirely. Although you may have been told you need red meat for its iron content, you can get all the iron you need from a multimineral tablet. You can still have white meat of chicken or turkey.

Fifth, you should consider giving up *fatty fish*, including salmon, trout, and catfish. These are high-fat, farm-fed fish that swim around fish ponds all day eating fishmeal. They don't swim a lot or catch other fish. They just get fat. If you can find ocean-caught salmon, buy it, as it is lower in fat. It is only available in some stores for part of the year, however. Most salmon you buy in stores is farm-fed. You can have any other white fish (halibut, swordfish, snapper, sea bass, scrod, cod, sole, ahi tuna, canned tuna in water, etc.). Shrimp, scallops, crabs, clams, and lobsters are OK as long as they are not deep-fried.

Sixth, consider minimizing your consumption of *cheese* and *cheese pizza*, or giving them up altogether. Cheese is between 60 and 80 percent fat. There are "fat-free" cheeses but these suffer from the same problem as fat-free margarine. Even "low-fat" cheese still has 70 percent of the fat found in real cheese. Besides, these are cheese foods, not cheese. If you want cheese on rare occasions, have some real cheese. It tastes good and your body will metabolize it. Just don't make it a regular part of your meals. Don't be fooled into thinking that you are adding protein to your turkey sandwich by adding a cheese slice. Most of the calories in cheese are from fat.

Last, consider minimizing or giving up desserts of *nonfat* and *low-fat yogurt*, and *ice cream*. They were never able to sell yogurt in this country until they made it taste like ice cream. The "fruit" they add has the equivalent of eight teaspoons of sugar, or about 130 refined sugar calories. Not only is there a lot of refined sugar that your body can turn into fat, but the eating behavior associated with nonfat yogurt is exactly the same as that associated with ice cream. It is a comfort food and a relaxing habit. So if you have a real craving for ice cream, walk to your neighborhood ice cream stand occasionally and have some. Just don't put it in your refrigerator where you can finish off a pint every evening. Try eating plain nonfat yogurt with slices of fresh fruit instead.

If this strategy seems impossible to follow, take heart. It's not that bad. Make each one of these steps a goal to work towards. It took me two years to give up pizza. I now eat pasta made with marinara sauce, which is a good substitute for the taste of pizza. I will sometimes order a cheese-less pizza, and I try to avoid the types of pizza crust doused and fried in oil.

An occasional splurge is fine. With this seven-step strategy, you will always know when you are on or off your diet without having to consult a dietitian and filling out a food record. You will get great results if you follow this plan 80 or 90 percent of the time. You don't have to be a fanatic.

Table 5.1. Diet Strategy by Food Groups

Choose	Decrease or eliminate
— Fish, Fowl, and Meats —	
White meat of chicken or turkey	Red meat, including veal, beef, pork, and lamb
Low-fat fish (swordfish, snapper, halibut, or canned tuna in water), shellfish	Salmon, trout, and catfish
— Dairy Products —	
Skim (nonfat) milk	Whole milk, 2% or 1% milk Evaporated and condensed milk

Choose	Decrease or eliminate
Fat-free cottage cheese	Nondairy creamers, whipped toppings
Sherbet, sorbet	Fat-free sour cream, fat-free cream cheese Ice cream, nonfat yogurts

— Eggs —

Egg whites (two egg whites for one egg)	Egg yolks

— Fruits and Vegetables —

Fresh fruits	Dried fruits Fruit juices
Fresh or steamed vegetables	Creamed vegetables or sauces as toppings

— Breads and Cereals —

Homemade baked goods using applesauce as an oil substitute	Commercial baked goods: cookies, doughnuts, pie, crackers, croissants
Rice, pasta	Egg noodles
Whole-grain cereals, breads	Breads in which cooking oil or eggs are a major ingredient
Homemade bread croutons with no oil	Commercial croutons

— Fats and Oils —

Baking cocoa	Chocolate
Roasted garlic as butter substitute	Butter, coconut, bacon fat

Choose	Decrease or eliminate
Natural fruit jam as spread or eat bread warm and steamy	Margarine or shortening Diet margarine
Wine vinegar with mustard	Low-fat and nonfat salad dressings
Rice vinegar with garlic	Dressings made with egg yolk or any salad oil, including so-called nonfat salad dressings
Mustard/relish	Mayonnaise, including so-called nonfat mayonnaise
Pretzels, air-popped popcorn	Seeds and nuts

TIPS FOR HEALTHY EATING THROUGHOUT THE DAY

For *breakfast*, try having a premeasured instant oatmeal or other high-fiber grain cereal and a full eight-ounce glass of nonfat milk along with half a grapefruit. Another breakfast could consist of two to three hard-boiled or poached egg whites seasoned with salsa or other spices. Avoid the yolk, since it contains the cholesterol and fat. Have your eggs with whole wheat bread and fruit jam. If you are one of those people who hates to eat breakfast, have a diet shake, such as Ultra Slim-Fast. In fact, you could keep a six-pack of the canned formulas in the back seat of your car. In case you forget a meal or get hungry on the road, drink a can. It beats pulling into a fast-food restaurant. Sometimes there is nothing open in town after I check in late at a hotel, so I take cans with me when I travel.

For *lunch,* I recommend a half to a full sandwich, depending on whether you are short or tall. Make it with high-fiber whole wheat bread and with tuna in water, white-meat chicken, or white-meat turkey. You can add mustard or relish, but no mayonnaise. For a change of pace, you can have a salad with meat slices on top. A piece of fruit is a flavorful and healthy dessert.

In the *midafternoon,* you should have fruit with a slice of high-fiber whole wheat or rye bread (if you are relatively short) or another diet shake (if you are tall and have a high metabolic rate). This afternoon snack will counteract that low-energy feeling many people get in the afternoon and make you less likely to overeat at dinner.

For *dinner,* imagine that your plate is made up of three different compartments about the sizes you would find in a frozen dinner. In the largest triangle, put either three ounces (shorter people) or six ounces (taller people) of white meat of chicken, turkey, white fish, shrimp, scallops, crab, clams, or lobster. In one of the smaller compartments, put one-half to one cup of rice, pasta, potatoes, beans, corn, or peas. In the other small compartment, put one cup of vegetables, such as carrots, asparagus, broccoli, Brussels sprouts, or string beans. Finally, fix a side dish of salad, without beans or croutons, dressed with wine vinegar, rice vinegar, or balsamic vinegar instead of salad dressing.

If you are still hungry *after dinner,* have some air-popped popcorn. Don't buy the prepackaged microwaveable popcorn you see at the store. Each package has a block of vegetable oil in it. Buy plain popcorn kernels instead and pop them in an air popper, which has a hot air blower that causes the water in each kernel to boil and pop the hull. While they don't taste as good as the prepackaged varieties, they are more filling per calorie than anything I have found. Don't buy the butter-flavored sprays for your popcorn, either. You will just be polluting your taste buds and making it harder to break your high-fat habits. The best thing to do after dinner is to walk out of the kitchen and get busy with something that will keep you from eating.

I have tried this diet strategy myself and taught it to doctors who have successfully used it with thousands of patients. It meets or exceeds the fat-reduction advice contained in most government guidelines. If you are eating less than 1,200 calories per day, you should also take a multivitamin/multimineral tablet and 1,000 mg of calcium with dinner. Women over the age of fifty should take an additional 500 milligrams of calcium per day to prevent osteoporosis. You should also take the other natural supplements that are discussed in Chapters 9 and 10.

HOW TO EAT WHEN YOU'RE OUT

Eating out has become a form of entertainment for most of us. Spurred on by gourmet cooks, restaurant critics, and restaurant advertising, we have converted the occasional treat of dining out into a way to either pass time on the weekend or grab a quick meal during the week.

When you eat out, you give control of your nutrition to the restaurant. It determines the portion size and the fat content of your meal. The portion size is usually large, so you will think you are getting a great value, and the fat content is usually high to enhance taste.

One of my patients was a famous restaurant critic on radio and television. He made his living tasting food at restaurants. He maintained a healthy weight and cholesterol level, and, with the exception of a weakness for champagne brunches, maintained a healthy diet. How? He simply didn't eat whole portions of anything. So you see, there are ways you can control the amount and quality of the food you eat by taking charge when you eat out. Let's look at ways to do so in different types of restaurants.

Fast Food

My recommendation is that you avoid fast food altogether. However, there will be times when it will be the only choice, especially if you've forgotten to carry a healthy snack (see page 65). These places usually have low-fat milk rather than nonfat milk, so your best choice is to avoid this usually good protein source. The fries are calling out to you in all their greasy glory. Avoid them. The burgers are a nutritional disaster area of fat and calories, so your best choice is a charbroiled chicken breast sandwich. This is called a BK Broiler at Burger King and a Broiled Chicken Breast Sandwich at Mac-Donald's and other chains. Avoid the deep-fried breaded chicken or fish, which are both loaded with oil. If you can get a garden salad, this is a good choice. Avoid eating too much dressing by dipping your fork in the dressing and then picking up your lettuce rather than pouring the dressing on top of your salad. Have a diet soda to complete your meal.

American Prepared Food

If you are willing to pay just a bit more, you can get much better food from a new variety of prepared food restaurants. Among these new chains are Boston Market and Kenny Roger's Roasters. One stands out in terms of healthy and delicious food. While not yet open in every part of the United States, Koo Koo Roo California Kitchens provides a flame-broiled chicken breast that has about 10 percent of its calories from fat. They also have steamed vegetables and fresh salads.

Chinese Food

Chinese food in China is among the lowest-fat foods in the world. It is high in fiber and rich in soy protein (see Chapter 10). Unfortunately, restaurants serving Chinese food in the United States have succumbed to American temptation, and now use fat in large amounts. As a result, Americanized Chinese food is among the highest-fat foods in the country.

So how can you stick to a healthy eating plan in a Chinese restaurant? Pass up the high-fat egg rolls, spareribs, and fried wonton dishes as appetizers and sip some green tea until the soup arrives. Egg-drop soup is made from egg whites and is fairly low in fat. A bowl of hot-and-sour soup is thickened with rice or corn starch. So far, so good.

Now comes the problem of portion control. Order steamed vegetables (broccoli, carrots, asparagus) and white rice (instead of fried rice). Then choose a dish made with Szechwan garlic sauce over white meat of chicken, shrimp, or scallops. Scallions add taste as well as healthy phytochemicals, substances that compete with dietary cholesterol for absorption into the bloodstream (see Chapter 9). Avoid dishes such as lemon chicken, Kung Pao chicken, orange duck or beef, and Hunan shredded pork. If you are particularly fond of these dishes, you may want to choose Chinese restaurants less frequently, or even avoid them altogether.

Italian and Greek Food

The traditional Mediterranean diets of Italy and Greece have a great reputation, since Italy and Greece had among the lowest rates of cancer and heart disease in the 1960s. This is where olive oil got its great reputation as the healthiest salad and cooking oil.

However, when Italian food was imported into the United States, cheese was added to pizza. Some pizza makers even stuff cheese into the crust, and others fry the pizza dough in cooking oil. In many Italian restaurants, oil and cheese are added to pasta dishes, or greasy meat sauces are used. Fettucine Alfredo, with its heavy cheese sauce is usually the highest fat and calorie choice on the menu. And unfortunately, diets in Italy have also become progressively higher in saturated fat and calories. As a result, the rates of heart disease and cancer have increased there, too.

To eat light at an Italian restaurant, order a traditional Italian salad (not the antipasto) with balsamic vinegar (no oil) on the side. Have no more than two slices of Italian bread. Order pasta with marinara sauce, and a shrimp, fish, or white-meat chicken dish. Ask them not to add oil to the order. Split the pasta, meat, and salad with a companion (usually the portions are large enough for two). This sharing policy not only cuts down on the size of the bill, but will cut the number of calories you consume. Pasta can make you fat, if you eat enough of it.

Greek salad is very similar to Italian salad except it is usually made with feta cheese. Again, ask for the dressing on the side. Beyond the salad, you have a problem. The lamb used for gyros is high in fat, so you may want to look for a white-meat chicken dish or a fish dish. If there is a vegetarian dish without cheese, that could be a good choice. Obviously, this isn't easy. If it's a special occasion, cut down on the high-fat main dish and have double helpings of salad and vegetables.

Japanese Food

There are some great choices available in Japanese restaurants, such as miso soup, sushi, and white rice.

Teriyaki made with white-meat chicken or shrimp is fine. Have wasabe mustard (careful, it's really hot), and be sure to avoid all tempura dishes, since they are deep-fried.

Mexican Food

Like Chinese food, Mexican food in the United States is high in fat, while Mexican food in Mexico is relatively healthy. Serving tortilla chips fried in oil is a shame, since they could as easily be baked without the oil. The oily kind provides about 500 calories per basket, so push away the basket of chips and salsa while you are waiting to order. Refried beans (frijoles) are made with lard or vegetable oil, which adds unnecessary fat and calories. There is usually shredded cheddar cheese in most dishes. Finally, margaritas are among the highest calorie drinks, delivering up to 350 calories per drink.

If you want a drink, a light beer with a slice of lemon is a good choice, and sparkling water with lime is even better. I usually order a chicken, fish, or shrimp tostada. I eat the meat and some of the lettuce. I will have some of the beans and pass on the cheese and the high-fat taco shell. An interesting alternative is ceviche. This is an appetizer made with seafood marinated in vinegar. If you can get whole black beans, they are a better choice than refried beans. Add lots of salsa, which is rich in tomatoes, onions, and cilantro, and eat hot peppers with your food. The general principle is to make your meals more interesting by substituting spice for fat.

HOW TO EAT WHEN YOU'RE HOME

You will be surprised at the togetherness that can come from preparing and sharing a meal with those you love. The dinner table used to be the place where everyone came together to share their day and discuss important family matters. Dinner can enrich family life at a time when family members are running in so many different directions.

No matter whether you are a naturally great cook, or can't boil water, it is possible today to combine healthy ingredients. By simply changing the way you shop and cook in little ways, you will be able to provide yourself and your family with a healthy, low-fat diet. I want to share some of the things I have found that are easy to do and help to cut fat.

Chicken Breasts

Buying precut, boneless chicken breast without skin from a supplier who uses no hormones or preservatives can provide a great start to one of the most versatile protein items you can prepare. You can marinate chicken breasts in a variety of sauces, including teriyaki marinade, Italian spices, and orange sauce. Serve with pasta and tomato sauce, or with rice, noodles, or potatoes. If you love to barbecue, chicken can be a great substitute for hamburger or steak. Be careful of turkey burgers made with dark meat. These can have up to 40 percent of their calories from fat, although they are labeled 22 percent fat by weight.

If you want to have a barbecue regardless of the weather outside, and if you have a gas stove, you can buy a nonstick cooktop broiler. The fat from the chicken drips down into a stainless steel trough at the base. These devices usually cost about twenty dollars, and are easy to clean. Cook extra chicken breasts for economical low-fat sandwiches.

Shrimp

Shrimp can be made on a skewer with red pepper,

green pepper, and onion slices. You can sauté shrimp with garlic or scallions, and put them over pasta or white rice. You can also add shrimp to a tomato sauce with garlic or mushrooms, and layer the sauce over pasta for a great gourmet meal. While shrimp is more expensive than other meats on a per-pound basis, you only need three to six small shrimp per person to meet the dinnertime protein requirement.

Fish

Ahi tuna, swordfish, and halibut are great barbecued. You may need to get a special basket to keep the fish from falling apart on the barbecue. You can also broil fish indoors on an elevated grill to separate the fish from the fatty drippings. Add scallions, soy sauce, or teriyaki sauce for variety. One of my other favorites is cioppino, or fisherman's stew. Simply put cut-up fish and tomato sauce with oregano, garlic, and other seasonings to taste in a big pot, and simmer. You can also add scallops and shrimp to make the cioppino restaurant style.

Vegetables

You get more micronutrients if you don't boil non-starchy vegetables in water. Steam vegetables such as broccoli, carrots, or asparagus in a double boiler or steamer. Or add a small amount of water to a covered microwave-safe dish, add the vegetables, and microwave for a few minutes. Don't add butter, salt, cheese, or oil. Instead, use seasonings such as rosemary, thyme, celery salt, dried onions, and dried garlic or garlic powder. Or mix different vegetables together for variety.

Potatoes are easy to bake in the microwave. Add salsa or plain nonfat yogurt as a sour cream substitute. Using beans and other legumes (peas, lentils, chickpeas, etc.)

is a great way to add protein value to vegetarian dishes. Use equal amounts of legumes and either corn or rice to provide a balanced serving of protein. Approximately one cup of beans and one cup of rice is equivalent to a four-ounce serving of chicken in protein. Be careful, though. When you add lots of beans to a meal, you also add significant calories.

Rice

Buy an electric rice cooker. These devices are inexpensive, easy to use and clean, and make great brown or white rice when used as directed. A rice cooker can be set to cook during the day, while you're out of the house. Make life easier with an automatic rice cooker and you will be able to include this low-fat carbohydrate in more of your dinners.

Pasta

There are many varieties of pasta, from angel hair to mostaciolli to ziti. Choose the shapes your family likes best. Then boil the pasta in a big pot until it is cooked through but still firm (al dente). One trick I learned from a local chef was to boil an extra pot of water. When you strain the pasta, rinse it once with the extra water just before serving. This will both heat up the pasta and remove the sticky gluten on the outside of the pasta that can make it pasty. Cover the pasta with the lowest-fat prepared pasta sauce you can find for an easy meal. For a different taste, cook spinach leaves and add crushed garlic to taste. Put this over the pasta after you ladle out the sauce.

Salads

Buy bagged lettuce that is already cut up. This eliminates the most labor-intensive part of making a salad.

The dark green types of lettuce, such as endive, chico-
ry, and escarole, have more micronutrients than watery
iceberg lettuce. Some dark lettuces taste like licorice,
while others have a slightly bitter taste. After the lettuce is in place, get a chopping board and go to town.
Add green pepper, red pepper, mushrooms, carrots, al-
falfa sprouts and anything else you want—just do not
add croutons or beans. Use flavored vinegar instead of
oil. You can buy rice vinegar in various flavors, red
wine vinegars, or balsamic vinegar. If you are eating because of stress, having seconds on salad is a great idea.

Desserts

Cut-up melon, such as honeydew, cantaloupe, and wa-
termelon, make a great summertime dessert. If available,
add some grapes and chopped pineapple. In the winter,
a nutless Waldorf salad made with apples, pears, raisins,
and cranberry juice is terrific. This salad can also be
cooked in the microwave and served warm.

Sorbets made from fruits such as strawberries or rasp-
berries are easy summer treats. Just add some fruit and
chopped ice to a blender. Blend until a slush forms,
scoop the mixture into dishes, and place the dishes in
the freezer. Serve with a sprig of mint and it will seem
to your guests that you have been reading the latest
gourmet cookbooks.

I hope you agree that my seven-step strategy is lot easier to understand than some of the more complicated
diet plans. I know that doesn't make it easy to follow.
Remember, it took you a lifetime to acquire the eating
habits you have now. Don't expect to change everything
overnight. Take it a step at a time, and go ahead and
splurge once in a while. I hope my tips for eating out
and at home help make following this strategy a little

easier. You will soon find yourself thinking of other ways to cut the fat out of your meals.

Why do people overeat? Many times, people don't eat out of hunger or for taste but simply to reduce stress. Boredom and stress are common reasons for adding extra calories and fat to the diet. The stress-diet connection is an important one, and it can sabotage your best intentions when it comes to changing your diet. The way to break this connection is to reduce your stress level and change your diet at the same time. In the next chapter, you will learn about healthy and unhealthy ways of reducing stress.

CHAPTER 6

Stress and Your Heart—
The Mind-Body Connection

S ome stress is good. Stress provides us with the ability to be alert to danger and to flee when necessary. It can stimulate us to do our best—great actors and actresses will tell you that they are often nervous when they give their best performances. (On the other hand, we have all seen children unable to deliver their lines in the class play because of stage fright.) The total absence of stress can actually be stressful. Just ask all those children who give the same plaintive refrain every summer: "I'm bored! There's nothing to do."

Yet while a certain level of stress is good, most of us have an excessive level of stress. Ultimately, this continuing stress can lead to the most common form of depression, called burnout depression. Stress can also contribute to an increase in both blood cholesterol levels and the risk of heart disease. In this chapter, I'll discuss stress and its effects on the body before going on to discuss methods of stress relief, both healthy and unhealthy.

THE STRESS CONTROL SYSTEM

Ancient humans had obvious stressors. A man would see a saber-toothed tiger and decide whether to fight (if it was a really small tiger and he had a club) or, more likely, to flee. The alertness needed to make this decision was provided by "fight or flight" hormones called *catecholamines*. These hormones make you feel nervous: your palms sweat, your pulse races, and your blood pressure rises.

Today, saber-toothed tigers have been replaced by more persistent stresses that you cannot run away from as easily. For example, newspaper writers who work against a daily deadline have terrible stress. This ultimately takes its toll, since these journalists have high rates of heart disease. In the extreme, stress can even stop your heart from beating. This occurs when someone is literally scared to death.

While modern society has brought us many technological innovations and labor-saving devices, it has also increased the amount of stress many of us feel. We all know the telltale signs, such as our stomachs becoming tied up in knots. There is pressure to compete and excel at every level, despite deadlines that seem to get shorter with each passing year. We can also feel anxiety about our ability to make the grade, as we strive to achieve standards (real or imagined) that are constantly on the rise. Despite the prediction twenty years ago that the Age of Automation would usher in a new era of relaxation and leisure, Americans now work harder than they ever have before. Our society does not put a high value on stress reduction on our highways, in our stores and malls, or at our jobs.

Often, however, we seem to be losing ground. We work longer hours, yet seem to be running in place. When one crisis passes, another seems to be right there to frustrate our best intentions. We can feel like rats in a maze. The end result: stress.

Excessive stress can contribute to a number of physical ailments, including headaches and stomachaches, ulcers, colitis, and high blood pressure. It can worsen pre-existing arthritis and asthma, and even result in sexual dysfunction.

Stress can also worsen heart disease. When we get nervous, our hearts beat faster. The rate at which the heart consumes oxygen also goes up. A heart attack occurs when the amount of oxygen the heart needs can no longer be delivered to the heart muscle. Yet when there are high levels of stress hormones in the body, the heart works less efficiently than when it is beating more slowly. This means it requires more oxygen to do the same amount of work. And as we'll soon see, stress can lead to a rise in cholesterol levels.

If you don't want stress to affect your health, you will have to learn to control it. When you are in control, the stress you feel will not take its terrible toll. There is a famous experiment I first heard about in my college psychology class that involved two monkeys. One was given food every time he pressed a lever after a green light went off. He got an electrical shock every time he pressed the lever after a red light flashed. The green and red lights went off in a predictable manner, and the monkey soon learned which lever to push. The other monkey was given a random sequence of green and red lights when each of the two levers was pushed. It was impossible to learn which lever to push, and the poor monkey ultimately developed a stress ulcer trying to figure it out. If the levers in your life are random and unpredictable, then you need to bring order to your life. Lifestyle changes can help. First let's see how stress and depression affect cholesterol levels.

STRESS, DEPRESSION, AND CHOLESTEROL

One of the ways in which stress promotes heart disease is through its influence on cholesterol levels. There are a number of studies that associate a rise in cholesterol levels with various types of emotional stress. School exams, occupational problems, the loss of a job, and surgery are common experiences that have caused stress for many of us. All of these situations can lead to increased total cholesterol levels and lowered levels of the good cholesterol, HDL. (For a complete discussion of cholesterol, see Chapter 4.) Let's look at some of these studies.

A study examined the cholesterol levels of accountants before, during, and after tax season. There was a direct correlation between the pressure they felt to beat the tax deadline of April 15 and their cholesterol levels. In fact, the cholesterol levels of the accountants in this study went up by 20 percent during tax season. Although diet was not considered in this study (a major oversight, since accountants often order fast food when working late), it is frequently quoted as an example of how stress affects cholesterol levels.

Another study conducted at the University of Michigan examined the impact of job loss on cholesterol levels. Two hundred married men with stable employment histories lost their jobs due to a plant closure. Their cholesterol levels were monitored for two years, during which most of the men found new jobs. The study found a direct relationship between unemployment and cholesterol levels. When the men were without work, their stress and cholesterol levels rose in tandem. Once they found gainful employment, both levels dropped in direct proportion. The researchers also found a correlation between cholesterol levels and depression.

There are forms of depression that are not stress-re-

lated. These disorders, which are caused by chemical im-
balances in the brain, are treated with therapy and
drugs. In most cases, however, depression is the result
of unrelenting stress. Stress-related depression, which is
called *burnout depression*, is due to a reduction in the
brain levels of a chemical known as serotonin. Genetic
factors also play a role.

As a physician who deals with nutritional problems,
I see many patients who have a mild form of depression called *dysthymia*. About one-quarter of all overweight patients seen in weight-reduction clinics have
this type of depression, which most commonly results
from a chemical imbalance brought on by too much
stress. Ten years ago, such patients were treated with
antidepressants that caused weight gain. More recently,
doctors have used a new class of antidepressants that
increased serotonin levels while causing weight loss.
Prozac was the first and most famous of these drugs.

Like dysthymia, burnout depression often occurs in
obese or overweight individuals who have a high total
cholesterol level, a low HDL level, and a high triglyceride level. It occurs commonly among diabetics, who
have similar levels of fat in the blood. For many people, eating sweets will lessen depression, especially in
those individuals who characterize themselves as "choco-
holics." How does sugar intake affect depression? An increase in sugar levels causes an increase in the level of
insulin, the chemical that regulates the amount of sugar
in the blood. An increase in insulin, in turn, causes an
increase in serotonin levels, which produces a pleasur-
able sensation. Thus, the woman who eats a pint of
chocolate ice cream after losing her boyfriend may be
doing something that counteracts her natural feelings of
depression. This is a good example of the connection
between the mind and the body.

The person who retains excess body fat is more likely than other people to be depressed. It is important to treat both problems together. The treatment for depression includes diet, exercise, and stress reduction, as well as medication. These are the same treatments we are recommending for everyone concerned with excessive cholesterol. So perhaps the prevention of depression is one benefit you will also obtain from reading this book. If you currently have depression, what we are recommending here can only help.

CIGARETTES AND ALCOHOL: UNHEALTHY METHODS OF STRESS REDUCTION

Different people relieve stress in different ways. Many patients attempt to deal with stress and depression not through exercise and stress reduction methods but through smoking and drinking. They believe that covering up their stress with these bad habits will somehow neutralize them. While there is some evidence that small amounts of alcohol may be beneficial in reducing stress, there is no such evidence for cigarettes.

Smoking, Stress, and Heart Disease

Cigarettes have clearly been linked to both heart disease and cancer in numerous studies. Cigarette smoke is a pro-oxidant, which means that it can promote atherosclerosis (see Chapter 4). It also affects the heart's blood circulation. Cigarette smoke not only harms the smoker, but can also affect the health of other people who inhale second-hand smoke.

You may be wondering about the stress reduction potential of cigarettes. After all, smokers feel relaxed after they inhale. However, this relaxation appears to be related to the temporary satisfaction of their nicotine craving. When the body is deprived of nicotine, it reacts very negatively. As with all other physically addictive substances, the body goes into withdrawal, which creates a variety of stress-producing responses. Once the smoker supplies his or her body with the requisite nicotine, these responses go away temporarily, resulting in a momentary period of relaxation.

Despite the sensation of relaxation, tobacco stimulates both the brain and the spinal cord, and the body as a whole. While alcohol depresses the functions of the body, tobacco accelerates them.

If you are a smoker, quitting makes good sense. The best way to quit is cold turkey. If you need help with the real withdrawal symptoms, there are nicotine patches or nicotine gums that you can use.

Social pressure is a very effective way to discourage smoking. In California, the rate of tobacco use dropped significantly in the 1980s. One of the big factors in this reduction was tax-supported advertising against smoking as well as restrictions on smoking in restaurants, airplanes, and other public places. The ads stressed the social problems of smoking, with an emphasis on stained teeth and bad breath. So if you do smoke, join the trend and quit.

Watch Your Alcohol Consumption

I was once flying to Washington, D.C. for a government meeting, and the plane was routed through Nashville. A man sat down next to me and started drinking small bottles of Tennessee whiskey that the stewardess had given him. At first, he was friendly and talkative. About two-thirds of the way through the flight, he became paranoid and said he didn't like my looks. As we were landing, he was just about to punch me when he passed out.

This progression of symptoms occurs with all anesthetics, and alcohol is an anesthetic. It can lead to violence. It deadens you to your real problems. So if you are having a fine glass of Chardonnay to enhance your meal or a light beer to accompany your football game on TV, enjoy. But if you are drinking to escape your problems, then you are making a mistake that can lead to real trouble.

Several decades ago, the Multiple Risk Factor Intervention Trial looked at a group of over 11,000 middle-aged men for seven years. The study showed that those who consumed two alcoholic drinks per day had higher HDL levels than those who did not drink. A drink was defined as twelve ounces of beer, four ounces of wine, or one and a half ounces of 80-proof hard liquor. Researchers also noted a 22 percent reduction in deaths from heart disease in the group that consumed alcohol compared with those who did not. They suggested that stress reduction rather than the alcohol itself caused the rise in HDL levels. A 1984 study noted that alcohol consumption had no effect on HDL levels for people who regularly participate in aerobic exercise.

The skin of grapes contains an antioxidant called resveratrol, which is found in red wine. It has been thought to be responsible for the French paradox: The French drink lots of wine and eat a high-fat diet, but have a lower incidence of heart disease than we do in this country. However, there are other factors involved. The portions served in France are smaller, and the French walk more than we do. So the lower rate of heart disease in France may be due to a combination of factors, including lower stress levels, exercise, and diet. You will no doubt hear that red wine prevents heart disease, but there's more to it than simply the effect of the antioxidants found in French wines.

There are some nutritional considerations that you also need to keep in mind. While alcohol is fat- and cholesterol-free, it is not calorie-free. Each gram of alcohol has seven calories. That's less than the nine calories per gram of fat, but more than the four calories in each gram of protein or carbohydrate. The calories of alcoholic drinks can be higher than you suspect due to the ingredients that are mixed with them. Piña coladas may have a great taste, but they contain coconut and cream, both of which add fat and calories. You may be surprised to know that a margarita can easily have over 350 calories. For the same reason, you want to avoid drinks made with ice cream. Specialty liquors, such as Irish and coffee creams, often contain milk or cream products that add calories. On the other hand, a light beer might be 90 to 110 calories and a glass of wine might provide about 100 calories. So the best choice from a dietary point of view would be a glass of wine or light beer rather than either hard liquor or a mixed drink.

If you want to engage in moderate alcohol consumption, go ahead. A drink or two per day isn't going to hurt you, and if it helps you melt away your stress, it may actually help. Keep in mind that there are many healthy ways that you can relax after a hard day's work. I want to make a clear distinction between having one or two drinks to relax on one hand and finishing a half bottle of wine or having five hard liquor drinks on the other. If reducing stress is your goal, there are options other than alcohol available to you. You could try tai chi, yoga, a jazz aerobics class, or a walk around the park.

If you don't already drink alcohol, I would not want alcohol's supposed health benefits to encourage you to start drinking. There are far better ways to get and keep a healthy heart. Find some recreational activity that you like and participate in it regularly. Feel your muscles pumping and delight in the wonderful relaxation that follows. You'll be able to feel the enjoyment with all of your senses intact. Of course, be sure to eat properly.

HEALTHY METHODS OF STRESS REDUCTION

There are many techniques you can use to bring relief from the anger, hostility, frustration, and stress that life's experiences can bring each of us from time to time. These techniques complement the dietary recommendations I made in Chapter 5. Together, these lifestyle enhancements will enable you to keep a lid on stress and help make life's journey as pleasant as possible.

The three main ways you can deal with stress are to:

• Reduce the total number of stressful situations

• Decrease the severity of each stressful episode

• Find ways to relax and refresh yourself between stressful episodes

Easier said than done, you say? Quite true. But it's well worth the effort. One of the reasons why so many people live their lives in a depressed or stressed-out state is because it's so easy to do so. Just react to all of the negative feedback life gives you, and you too can be anxious and unhappy! You need to follow a different path, one that will have much greater rewards. Accept the challenge of helping your heart to perform its essential task by making a personal effort to stamp out stress. You'll live longer and enjoy it more.

The first task is to get in touch with your own feelings. What causes you stress? Different situations bring varying levels of stress to different people. Some persons are able to handle high stress levels with minimal problems, while others fly apart at the slightest provocation. Keep a diary of the events that produce stress for you. Then analyze each of them to see how you could alter the situation or at least change the way you respond to it. If you feel stress waiting in line at the bank, ask the teller when the bank isn't busy and rearrange your schedule to go at that time. If your schedule is restricted, at least bring a book or newspaper to pass the time while you work your way up the line. You'll be talking to the teller before you know it.

This method works for most stressful situations. If you're stressed by traffic, try leaving a bit earlier so you aren't constantly rushed. You could also listen to a soothing music station on the radio or bring relaxing CDs or cassettes to play on the way to work. A more radical solution would be to carpool. This would reduce the number of days you drive each week and should lower your stress level, provided you enjoy the people you're riding with!

The most difficult thing for many people is learning to relax. In modern society there are going to be some stressful situations. That is an unfortunate fact of life today. We can't retreat to the "good old days" and most people probably wouldn't want to anyway. Our only option is to learn to relax in the limited time we have available. It doesn't do any good to stew about something that made you angry and anxious. What's done is done. Put it behind you and use that time to create a relaxing moment you can enjoy and remember.

There are as many ways to relax as there are people. It may be a cliché to tell you to stop and smell the roses, but it can be effective if you enjoy flowers. You could also take a few minutes to take in a beautiful sunset. Counting to ten in a stressful situation may also work.

Most of us, however, need more structured forms of relaxation therapy. Fortunately, there are quite a few available. In addition to the many different types of exercise, there is yoga, tai chi, meditation, and several other Eastern disciplines that can help you achieve a more relaxed approach to life. Courses in these methods are offered in all metropolitan areas, and everyone can learn about these therapies through books and tapes. For people who need a bit more help in relaxing, group-analysis sessions and biofeedback training can be helpful.

One of the best ways to get rid of stress is also one of the most enjoyable: do something nice for yourself. Our society places such a high value on work that sometimes we forget that play is important, too. Working your fingers to the bone may be necessary at times for economic reasons, and it may have some spiritual value if you believe in the work ethic. However, all work and no play is no fun. It's also a great recipe for stress and depression in the long term. That special thing you do doesn't have to involve a major expenditure such as going on a world cruise, either. Little things are just as effective. Get a massage, or sneak away to that secret hiding place that only you know about. Try a steam bath or sauna, or perhaps a facial or manicure. The choice should be individual, since only you know what you really want. Whatever that is, do it, even if it's only for a few minutes out of a busy day. When you look back on your week, chances are that you will remember those precious moments more than all the work you did. And why not? Sometimes even reminiscing about a pleasant experience in your past will cause your stress levels to drop.

Finally, take a good look at your attitude. The way you approach life has a big impact on your life experiences. Perception can become reality. If you go through life thinking that the glass is half-empty, then for you it will be. If you wake up expecting the worst, then chances are it will happen. Wouldn't that be stress-producing! Why not look at the glass as being half-full, and expect good things to happen until you know otherwise? While these attitudes often develop in childhood and have deep roots, they can be changed. True, it does require both willpower and an open mind, but you can change your perceptions. In time, your reality will also change.

Don't think of life as one disaster following another, even if it sometimes feels that way. It's all in your attitude. If there are no parking spaces near the store you want to shop in, don't fret. Park a block or two away and use the time to get to know your neighborhood better. Do some window shopping, or chat with a friend you meet along the way. If a business associate is late for a meeting, don't sit there fuming. Make a few personal phone calls, or read that magazine that has been sitting in your in-basket for weeks on end. Facing a rainy weekend after five gorgeous, sunny days you only saw through your office window? Don't go crazy. Nature does not hate you. Explore that new museum or art gallery, or take in that movie you've been meaning to see but never seemed to have time for. It all works out in the end. When you approach life with a balanced, positive attitude, you can do your heart a world of good.

Face it! You live in a high-stress society. If you are to survive our modern-day saber-toothed tigers, you need to adapt. For years, I have been telling my patients about *The Seven Habits of Highly Effective People* by Steven Covey and his more recent work, *First Things First*. These books contain principles that can help you define what your goals are, and how you want to achieve these goals. Once you know your mission in life, you can prioritize those things that are most important and most urgent. Then you will learn to be in control of your own life, instead of giving that control to others.

You control how you respond to the stressful situations that life hands you. It's your life. And your heart. The choice seems clear.

In the early part of the twentieth century, psychiatrists in Central Europe came up with the concept of separation of mind and body. This led to the idea that there are separate physical and psychiatric illnesses. We now know that this notion is simplistic at best. The mind and body are connected as one. It is not a coincidence that some men who made work the central focus of their lives die within a year after retirement, or that an elderly individual often dies soon after the death of his or her spouse.

There is much that we don't know about the mind, but we do know that it can stop the heart's function as a result of intolerable fright. Years of chronic stress can also damage the heart, slowly but just as surely. Smoking and drinking along with the stress worsen the situation. So balance your life with the good guys—exercise and relaxation—and get rid of the bad guys—stress, depression, tobacco, and alcohol. You'll make your heart happy and healthy.

In the next chapter, we'll look at exercise. It can not only help to reduce stress, but can do other good things for your heart.

CHAPTER 7

What to Do When You Feel the Urge to Exercise

(Hint: Don't Wait Till It Passes)

One of the best ways to reduce stress and depression is to engage in physical exercise. Exercise holds the key to a more relaxed and balanced outlook on life, which improves your cholesterol profile (the ratio of good to bad cholesterol in your blood) and helps you to live longer. You don't have to become a marathon runner to receive benefits from exercise. Even moderate activity, such as regular walks in the park, can elevate your HDL level while lowering your total cholesterol level. (For an explanation of these terms, see Chapter 4.) So there's no reason why you can't squeeze a little exercise into your busy daily schedule. Once you get into the habit, I'm sure you'll discover that you feel better about yourself and about life in general.

There is another important part to the exercise equation. When you exercise, you increase your muscle mass. This boosts your body's ability to burn fat as well as sugar. The food in your diet is either burned for energy or stored as body fat. The more active you are and the more muscle you have, the more calories that are burned rather than stored. Muscle activity also tends to lower cholesterol levels, while the increased movement of blood through the veins within your muscles helps the heart do its job of pumping blood.

In this chapter, we'll first look at the benefits of exercise. We'll then look at how you can start an exercise program.

THE MAIN BENEFITS OF EXERCISE

Exercise benefits the body in many different ways. Among the most important benefits are:

- Better cholesterol profile

- Weight loss

- Stress reduction

These benefits result from two general types of exercise. *Aerobic training* benefits the heart and circulation directly by exercising the heart muscle. In aerobic training, you perform an activity at a great enough intensity that you attain your target heart rate for thirty minutes at least three times a week (see "Calculating Your Heart Rate" on page 98). Aerobic exercise can be anything that gets your heart going, from walking or running to gardening or swimming. As you can see, you don't need to pursue a sport to get aerobic exercise. Any leisure-time physical activity that is vigorous enough to stimulate your heart will suffice. You don't have to overdo it, either. It is estimated that one American in every four is totally sedentary, and that one in two is insufficiently active. Even a moderate amount of aerobic exercise would help these people.

The other general type of exercise is *resistance training*. Resistance training, such as weightlifting, benefits the muscles and bones. It does so by actually injuring the muscles, but in a way that forces the body to build even more muscle to repair the damage. The bigger and stronger muscles, in turn, put a strain on the bones and joints, which makes the bones stronger. Since we all tend to lose muscle as we age, due to both inactivity and the aging process itself, resistance training can maintain good physical functioning throughout our lives. It can also help prevent osteoporosis, or thinning of the bones.

The benefits of exercise interact. Studies have shown that when patients with high cholesterol levels are asked to exercise, it is often impossible to separate the benefits that result from increased physical activity, increased muscle mass, and weight loss from the psychological benefits. Each of these benefits can directly or indirectly reduce cholesterol levels.

While it has traditionally been assumed that only aerobic training can provide cardiovascular benefits, new research has shown that resistance training can improve cholesterol profiles. Building up muscle through weight training leads to an increase in the enzymes that burn fat and sugar within the muscle fibers, resulting in lower blood cholesterol levels. Think of the enzymes as the body's spark plugs. You need both gasoline and air to make an engine run, but it's the spark plug that gets the gas and air to ignite.

Exercise also triggers a series of actions within the body that boosts the effectiveness of an enzyme called lipoprotein lipase. This enzyme helps break down the triglycerides in your bloodstream, lowering their concentration over time. My studies, involving hundreds of men and women, have shown a clear relationship between losing weight and lowering cholesterol levels.

Weight loss is an additional exercise benefit. (Actually, it's the reason most people start an exercise routine.) As we've seen, when you lose weight or cut your caloric intake, you lower your cholesterol levels. When you exercise, you force your body to burn calories. The exact amount of calories burned depends on the activity you're involved in. However, all forms of exercise require the body to use either glucose (blood sugar) or body fat as an energy source. Unless you eat more to compensate, the end result will be a reduction in the amount of fat stored in your body. This can give you a more slender, toned, and muscular physique while also lowering your cholesterol levels.

Another major benefit of exercise is stress reduction. When you work out, you take your mind off the problems that have been annoying you all day. Exercise provides a safety valve for your stress levels, so you don't always feel as if you're living in a pressure cooker. True, you can carry your problems onto the playing field or jogging trail, but even if the escape is not complete you still get a healthy dose of stress reduction. Your heart knows the difference!

How does exercise reduce stress? Physical activity releases morphinelike substances called *endorphins* into your brain and bloodstream. As a result, things that would normally send you flying off the handle will not bother you as much if you start exercising regularly. You just have to make the effort to get to the gym or recreation area. The hardest part is that first step. Once you begin exercising, your stress will melt away. Many people who exercise say they finish with more energy than they started with. Even a few hours of relaxation will rejuvenate your spirits and send your stress level plummeting. The resulting increase in your HDL cholesterol will help keep your cardiovascular system in good working order. (For more information on the connection between stress and cholesterol levels, see Chapter 6.)

Exercise has a number of other benefits. A study at the University of California proved that exercise promotes the growth of collateral blood vessels. These vessels are able to supply some of the necessary blood to the heart muscle after clotting shuts down a main artery. This study examined eighteen pigs with closed-off coronary arteries. Nine of the animals were exercised on a treadmill, while the other nine remained sedentary. After five months, the animals that exercised showed twice the growth in collateral vessels compared with that seen in the sedentary pigs. This is great news for human heart patients, since a well-developed system of collateral vessels can reduce the probability of death from heart disease.

Another study examined dogs that had previously had heart attacks. Half of the dogs were exercised, while the other half were not. After six weeks, all of the dogs were tested on a treadmill to measure improvements in their cardiac function. None of the dogs that exercised showed any signs of a weak or poorly functioning heart, while seven of the eight sedentary dogs had cardiac arrhythmias (heartbeat irregularities) or other abnormalities. Yet another study shows that swimming reduces high blood pressure. Therefore, it appears that exercise helps repair a damaged circulatory system, allowing it to perform its essential function with greater efficiency.

Exercise also slows down your heart rate when you are not exercising. That is because physical activity strengthens the heart muscle, enabling it to pump more blood with each beat. While the average person's heart rate is seventy-two beats per minute, conditioned athletes can have rates as low as fifty beats per minute. A slower, conditioned heart is better able to respond to stressful and unexpected situations while using less oxygen, which can be life-saving in emergencies.

You don't have to be a competitive athlete to benefit from exercise. Researchers have discovered that even moderate exercise reduces your risk of heart disease.

The Multiple Risk Factor Intervention Trial studied the impact of exercise on more than 12,000 middle-aged men. It concluded that leisure-time physical activity, such as gardening, is a significant factor in reducing the incidence of heart disease. After seven years, this study found that people who engaged in moderate exercise had 37 percent fewer fatal heart attacks than persons who were sedentary. Another study looked at some 4,000 men aged thirty to sixty-nine. Researchers found that the men with low levels of physical fitness had a higher risk of death from cardiovascular causes than their peers who exercised, even when age and other factors were taken into account.

GETTING STARTED ON AN EXERCISE PROGRAM

All right. I know you think that "exercise" is a dirty word.

Your memories of running laps and doing jumping jacks in high school won't go away. I went to a high school where the matches of our chess and debate team drew bigger audiences than some of our athletic events. Our football team had a perfect record: 0 and 8. Our school administrators were wise to hire former professional football team players and ex-Marines as gym teachers. I probably owe a good part of my health to those dedicated teachers. I was pushed, cajoled, and forced to climb poles, jump sidehorses, and run a mile. All of these experiences gave me a healthy respect for the positive side of physical fitness.

Nowadays, many children play video games instead of the physically active childhood games of yesterday. It is part of an overall pattern. We park as close to the mall as we can before moving up and down on escalators while munching hot dogs. In short, as a society we have failed to organize our physical environment in a way that encourages normal physical activity, much less regular exercise.

You've seen the ads for treadmills, weights, and exercise machines of every description. Maybe you have one. However, these machines don't benefit you by collecting dust. You have to use them. So what is the key to getting the right amount of exercise? Is it technique? Endurance? No. It's simply making up your mind that you are going to exercise.

Exercise is the only healthy addiction. I have sometimes been so tired that I just couldn't face going to the gym for a workout. However, once I began working out on the stationary bike, my mood improved and I would have one of my best workouts ever. This was not just a figment of my imagination. The exercise had released endorphins, which influenced the pleasure center in my brain.

You can become addicted to the feeling of a good workout, too. Exercise is also an important tool in combating burnout depression, a common form of depression caused by stress (see Chapter 6). When you exercise, especially outdoors, your brain chemistry changes to fight the blue feelings. I have had friends who have taken up jogging after painful divorces. To this day, they claim that the habit saved them from despair.

Your aerobic workouts can be done up to seven days per week and should take forty minutes. Work up to your target rate during a ten-minute warm-up, maintain your target heart rate for twenty minutes, and cool down for ten minutes. You can do this on a treadmill or stationary bike while watching television. Try to do it every day, if you can. Another way to increase your aerobic fitness is to take a full day out for cycling or hiking on a weekend. You will feel the positive, relaxing effects of this exercise for a full day afterwards. Your heart will appreciate it, too.

Calculating Your Heart Rate

You should run, walk, or cycle at a pace that allows you to comfortably carry on a conversation. The heart rate that allows you to do this is called the *target heart rate*. This is the rate at which your heart is beating fast enough to become stronger by creating positive changes in the heart muscle.

You can easily check your own heart rate by placing a finger on the carotid artery in your neck. That's the one you can feel beating near your windpipe. Just count the number of beats for fifteen seconds and multiply by four.

Before calculating your target rate, you should check your *resting heart rate*. Check your resting rate after a full night's sleep, before you get out of bed. The faster the rate, the harder your heart has to work even before you start doing anything. Over time, your resting rate will drop as you become more physically fit.

You can calculate your target rate as follows:

1. Start by subtracting your age from the number 220. This is called your maximum heart rate (MHR):

$$220 - age = MHR$$

2. You now want to determine your initial target heart rate (ITHR). This is the heart rate you want to aim for during the first six weeks of your exercise program.

$$MHR \times .5 \text{ to } .6 = ITHR$$

3. After six weeks, your heart will be in better condition. You can then exercise at your conditioned target heart rate (CTHR), which is:

$$MHR \times .7 \text{ to } .8 = CTHR$$

For example, if you are fifty, your MHR is 170 and your ITHR would be 85 to 102 beats per minute. After you are accustomed to exercise, you can raise your exercise intensity to the CTHR, which would be 119 to 136 beats per minute. Always stay within these ranges, except when you are warming up and cooling down from exercise. If you drop below 50 percent of your maximum heart rate, you will be spending more time exercising than you need to while giving your heart less of a workout than it would like. Anything over 80 percent of the maximum rate is too intense. So stay within the appropriate range.

Building muscle through resistance training is also important. Each pound of muscle burns fourteen calories per day. That doesn't sound like much, but adding twenty pounds of muscle can boost the amount of energy you burn every day by almost 300 calories. This will allow you to eat more while maintaining your current body weight or, if you prefer, you can keep your food intake steady and lose body fat more quickly.

In order to build muscle, you must carefully stress your muscle fibers. While this causes microscopic damage to the fibers, the muscle overcompensates and as part of the repair process becomes stronger. This repair process involves so-called *satellite cells*, which develop as the result of chemical messages released from the damaged muscle fibers. The satellite cells then fuse with the damaged fibers. This leaves the muscle stronger and bigger, provided that you rest long enough to allow the muscle to rebuild and grow. This means you should wait about one to two days between resistance workouts on the same muscle.

It is also important to select exercises that work the muscles on both sides of a joint, such as the biceps and triceps in the upper arm. These pairs of muscles, called agonists and antagonists, work in opposition to each other. For example, when the biceps muscle is contracted, the triceps muscle is stretched, and vice versa. Exercising both muscles helps to balance the joint and prevent injury. Be sure to perform your exercises carefully, using a slow, controlled motion throughout the entire movement. Also, proper breathing is important. Breathe out as you lift or push the weight, and breathe in as you relax the muscle.

You should balance the time devoted to building strength and endurance in each muscle group. This can be accomplished by varying the number of sets of each exercise from three to seven and varying the number of repetitions in each set from eight to fifteen. You should vary the pace of the exercise as well, starting out at four to six seconds per repetition and speeding it up to two to three seconds per repetition when using higher weights and fewer repetitions. You should also get some instruction from a knowledgeable trainer. If you have any physical problems, see your doctor *before* beginning your exercise program.

A SCHEDULE FOR RESISTANCE TRAINING

The most important thing when building muscle is to not become discouraged. This is a gradual process that takes many months. Here is a sample schedule I have developed to let you gradually work your way into muscle building. Always ask a knowledgeable trainer how to use the various machines and exercise equipment at your gym. On your own, you might injure yourself or become discouraged.

Be sure to stretch all your muscle groups before lifting weights. Simple stretching techniques are taught by most exercise instructors and physical therapists.

Week 0

Get in the habit of going to the gym. Ask an exercise instructor or physical therapist to show you how to use the equipment. Don't worry about making progress, but be sure to develop a written plan for the exercises you plan to pursue.

Week 1

Three sets of fifteen repetitions (reps) per exercise. If you cannot do this number of reps, reduce the weight until you can. Also, don't jerk the weights rapidly. Instead, spend four to six seconds performing each rep. Mentally concentrate on the muscles you are using to get the maximum benefit. Rest thirty seconds between sets.

Week 2

Increase to five sets of fifteen reps per exercise. The last four reps of each set should cause a slight burning sensation in the muscles being trained.

Week 3

Increase to seven sets of fifteen reps per exercise.

Week 4

Decrease to three sets of twelve reps per exercise, but increase the weight so you give your muscles the maximum stimulus.

Week 5

Do five sets of twelve reps per exercise at this new weight.

Week 6

Do seven sets of twelve reps per exercise at the same weight.

Week 7

Do three sets of eight reps per exercise, but increase the weight again. Reduce the amount of time you take for each rep to two to three seconds. Rest forty-five seconds between sets.

Week 8

Do five sets of eight reps per exercise at this new weight.

Week 9

Do seven sets of eight reps per exercise at the same weight.

Week 10

Repeat Week 1 of the program. Of course, now that you have built new muscle, you will be stronger than you were the first time. Follow the same routine of sets and repetitions, but this time use more weight. This progressive resistance will shape and tone your muscles while increasing your strength.

Remember to start slowly, but start to exercise as soon as you can. Aerobics can be done every day in a number of ways, from a jog in the park to a ride on a stationary bike. Then start a resistance training program. Although muscle building is a long-term goal, your heart will start getting in better shape right away. So develop your personal exercise program and get the advice you need. You can build muscle at any age. Exercise will lower your cholesterol and triglyceride levels while improving your quality of life. What are you waiting for? Go for it!

In the next chapter, I'll discuss the prescription drugs that are used to reduce cholesterol levels.

CHAPTER 8

Are Drugs the Answer?

You may be wondering why there is a chapter on prescription drugs in a book that deals with natural remedies for a healthy heart. Well, there are several reasons. First, you may be taking one of these medications yourself or you may know family members who are taking them. You may discover that the side effects you or those you love have experienced are not unique. Second, you can't make an informed decision without all of the facts. You need to know about these drugs so you can clearly weigh the benefits and drawbacks of alternative natural products. That way you can become an enlightened medical consumer and take an active role in preserving your health and longevity.

In this chapter, I'll first provide an overview of prescription drugs. I'll then discuss some of the more widely used cholesterol-lowering drugs.

PRESCRIPTION DRUGS AND SIDE EFFECTS

When diet and exercise by themselves cannot lower cholesterol and triglyceride levels to acceptable ranges, doctors frequently recommend prescription drugs. (For a discussion of cholesterol and triglycerides, see Chapter 4.) These drugs work in a variety of ways to reduce the amounts of these substances in your body. Some of these drugs are moderately effective, while others can be very effective in certain instances. All drugs have side effects, however. In some cases, the side effects are modest and considered an acceptable price to pay for the benefits received from the medication.

What is a drug? A drug is a substance that is either artificially synthesized or derived from a natural product through the isolation of some chemical building block. The pharmaceutical industry isolates these substances in an effort to maximize potency and minimize toxic effects. (*Potency* is defined by tests measuring a drug's ability to do such things as lower cholesterol or fight bacteria.) A famous example of a chemically manipulated natural product is the birth control pill. In the late 1940s, it was impossible to synthetically make the various hormones needed for birth control pills. Dr. Carl Djerassi, working in Mexico City at the time, found that the Mexican yam had a chemical that could be used as the building block for the creation of birth control pills.

Sometimes, though, that building block is the source of both the drug's effectiveness and its side effects. For example, digoxin, a drug used to strengthen the heart, is derived from foxglove. The foxglove plant contains a chemical that causes the human heart to increase its contractions. It is believed that this same chemical causes the natural predators of the foxglove to keep their distance. Foxglove can actually cause birds that eat it to get sick. So it's not surprising that in humans, the side effects of digoxin include nausea.

The U.S. Food and Drug Administration began to regulate drugs in the 1930s, after several deaths occurred because of a contaminated antibiotic. The contamination episode led to a national campaign, headed by Eleanor Roosevelt, to regulate the pharmaceutical industry. Since that time, the public's response to the famous thalidomide birth defects of the 1960s and other horror stories have helped to keep in place a very expensive but carefully monitored system to protect the public from the side effects of drugs. This has raised the cost of drug treatments, but has also helped to stimulate the development of the finest health-care system in the world.

In pharmaceutical laboratories, natural products are treated chemically to "remove impurities." When I talk to some medicinal chemists about natural products such as herbs, they say that these are simply mixtures of some active drugs and a lot of impurities. However, it is those "impurities" that can often reduce an herb's side effects. Natural products are usually mixtures of several substances with different actions that often work together to produce a better effect with less toxicity. This is why Congress passed the Dietary Supplement and Health Education Act, which exempts natural products from the lengthy and costly process required of pure prescription drugs.

Whenever you use a drug—or a natural product, for that matter—it is important to weigh the risks and benefits. When a disease poses a risk such as that posed by advanced cancer, let's say, the drug-induced side effects pale in comparison with the need to pull out all the stops in treating the disease. Therefore, this book is not targeted at patients with advanced heart disease. In such patients, drugs may well make sense along with surgery and other drastic measures. This book is aimed at people with high cholesterol levels who *do not yet* have serious heart disease, as well as at people with normal cholesterol levels who simply want to keep their hearts healthy.

It is important to remember that no therapy, natural

or synthetic, will work without cooperation from the patient. That means the patient must not only take the medicine according to directions, but must also make the necessary changes in lifestyle. For example, I have worked extensively with weight-loss drugs over the past few years. I have found that these drugs have the best effect in patients who also follow a healthy diet and make other lifestyle changes. Some patients think they can take the pills and eat whatever they want, but they are rarely successful. I have found that the patients who forget to take their diet pills are also the ones who forget to follow their diet. The effects of these drugs are best seen when they are taken by individuals who make positive lifestyle changes at the same time.

CHOLESTEROL-LOWERING PRESCRIPTION DRUGS

There are three main types of cholesterol medication currently in use: bile-acid sequestrants, fibrates, and HMG-CoA reductase inhibitors. There is another drug called probucol, which is chemically unrelated to the others. Niacin (vitamin B_3) is sometimes considered a drug when used to lower cholesterol levels because of the dosages required for it to be effective. However, we will look at the role of niacin in Chapter 10, which covers products that are available without a prescription.

Bile-Acid Sequestrants

There are two medications in this class: colestipol (Colestid) and cholestyramine (Questran, Questran Light). First developed in the 1960s, both of these drugs are powders that function within the intestinal tract. They are never absorbed by the body. Colestipol and cholestyramine are usually taken as two scoops twice a day in juice or yogurt.

Bile acids help digest fat. The liver uses cholesterol to create bile acids, which are released into the intestines by way of the gallbladder. Bile-acid sequestrants soak up these cholesterol-laden bile acids in a spongelike action. This keeps the cholesterol from moving through the intestinal wall for transport to the bloodstream. Instead, these chemically bound bile acids pass through the intestines until they are eliminated in the stool. This forces the body to produce more bile acids in order to make up the deficit. It does so by converting additional cholesterol to bile acids in the liver. Over time, this reduces the amount of cholesterol circulating in the bloodstream.

Since the body responds to the loss of bile acids by increasing its production of cholesterol, the net reduction in cholesterol levels with bile-acid sequestrants is less than with the HMG-CoA reductase inhibitors discussed on pages 111 to 113. However, the two types of drugs can be used in combination to achieve a greater combined effect because each drug works through different mechanisms.

Bile-acid sequestrants do lower total cholesterol and LDL cholesterol levels, although they are not effective in reducing triglyceride levels. The average drop in total cholesterol is 10 percent, while LDL cholesterol drops by 10 to 20 percent. Colestipol and cholestyramine can also raise HDL cholesterol by 3 to 8 percent. To get these benefits, you would need to take 20 to 30 grams of colestipol or 16 to 24 grams of cholestyramine per day.

Gastrointestinal side effects in the upper tract include indigestion, heartburn, burping, and a feeling of fullness, if not bloating. Problems in the lower tract include gas and diarrhea or constipation (depending on the foods you eat), as well as a greater quantity of bowel movement. These drugs cannot be used in patients with severe constipation without the use of additional medications to address the constipation.

Colestipol and cholestyramine can also interfere with the absorption and effectiveness of other drugs that may be prescribed. Cholestyramine, as an example, interacts with warfarin, a drug used to prevent clotting of the blood, and with the thiazide diuretics, which help to control high blood pressure. These and other fat-soluble drugs and vitamins should not be taken at the same time as bile-acid sequestrants. To avoid interference with absorption, the other drugs should be taken either one hour before or four to six hours afterwards.

Fibrates

There are two drugs in the fibrate family: gemfibrozil (Lopid) and clofibrate (Atromid-S). Both of these medications are chemically related to each other, but for some reason gemfibrozil has a much better track record than clofibrate.

Gemfibrozil works by reducing the production of VLDLs in the liver, which has the effect of lowering LDL levels in the blood. (For an explanation of why this happens, see Chapter 4.) It also causes a moderate increase in HDL levels at the recommended dosage of 1,200 milligrams (1.2 grams) per day. A 1987 Finnish study found that gemfibrozil lowered total cholesterol and LDL cholesterol levels by 8 percent, while HDL cholesterol levels increased by 10 percent. Triglyceride levels dropped by 35 percent.

The downside of these reduced concentrations of LDL and total cholesterol in the bloodstream is that cholesterol levels rise in the liver when this medication is used. That is because gemfibrozil keeps the liver from manufacturing VLDLs and shipping them out into the blood, so there is more "raw material" left inside the liver. This excess cholesterol can even lead to the development of gallstones, which may require gallbladder surgery.

Because of these negative side effects, persons with impaired liver and kidney function or those with a pre-existing gallbladder condition should *never* use gemfibrozil. For people without these conditions, side effects tend to be infrequent. When they occur, they often affect the gastrointestinal tract, causing diarrhea, flatulence, nausea, and abdominal pain. Occasional adverse reactions can include dizziness, headaches, insomnia, anemia, muscle pain, rashes, blurred vision, and ringing in the ears.

Clofibrate is rarely used anymore. While it usually lowers LDL levels by stopping production of the VLDLs, it sometimes causes an elevation of LDL concentrations in the bloodstream. Even when it does work, the reductions in LDL cholesterol tend to be modest. The death blow for clofibrate was a 1978 World Health Organization study that showed significant increases in death rates among users of the drug. There is no indication that gemfibrozil shares this danger despite its chemical similarity to clofibrate.

HMG-CoA Reductase Inhibitors

HMG-CoA reductase inhibitors are the newest family of anticholesterol drugs. First introduced in the United States in 1987, this type of medication works inside the liver by reducing the body's own production of cholesterol. As I noted in Chapter 4, HMG-CoA reductase is an essential enzyme, or catalyst, for the manufacture of cholesterol. These drugs work by blocking the action of this enzyme. With this source of production stopped, the body meets its needs for cholesterol by absorbing greater amounts from the bloodstream. The net result is a decline in blood levels of LDL cholesterol.

There are currently five medications in the HMG-CoA

reductase inhibitor category: lovastatin (Mevacor), fluvastatin (Lescol), pravastatin (Pravachol), simvastatin (Zocor), and atorvastatin (Lipitor). This class of drugs is also referred to as the *statins*. They share many characteristics but are not necessarily interchangeable. A doctor's final decision on which of them to use may depend on the side effects associated with each. Or it may depend on the doctor's familiarity with the various statins. Lovastatin and simvastatin are very similar in chemical structure and properties.

On average, LDL cholesterol levels are reduced by 30 to 40 percent with full doses of pravastatin (40 mg/day), simvastatin (40 mg/day), and lovastatin (80 mg/day). Fluvastatin is entirely synthetic and the least expensive of the statins, but it is also the least potent. Full doses of fluvastatin (80 mg/day) lower LDL cholesterol levels by 25 to 35 percent. Declines in triglyceride levels range from 10 to 30 percent. Increases in HDL cholesterol range from 2 to 15 percent.

Statins can also reduce the death rate from advanced heart disease. One Scandinavian study found that simvastatin reduced overall mortality from heart disease compared with a placebo (an inert substance used for comparison purposes). Another trial, the Cholesterol and Recurrent Events Study in Scotland, demonstrated that pravastatin lowered total mortality in men with no history of heart disease. Atorvastatin has been shown to lower both cholesterol and triglyceride levels.

These drugs can be very effective, but as with all drugs they have side effects. The most common are insomnia, fatigue, muscle aches, headaches, nausea, and skin rashes. The HMG-CoA reductase inhibitors can also elevate the levels of other essential liver enzymes. These enzyme concentrations can jump to more than three times their normal ranges in up to 2 percent of users, although there are often no noticeable symptoms associated with the changes. These variations are dose-dependent—the higher the dose, the more often the enzyme elevations are noted. Because of these potential difficulties, it is recommended that patients on these drugs have blood tests every two to three months for the first six to twelve months. After that, a blood test every three to four months should be sufficient. Persons with liver disease or any unexplained rise in their liver enzyme levels should *avoid* use of these medications entirely, as should women of childbearing age.

The statins can also produce inflammation of the muscles. While this is quite rare when these drugs are used alone, the incidence of inflammation increases when the HMG-CoA reductase inhibitors are used in conjunction with other cholesterol medicines such as gemfibrozil (Lopid; see page 110) and niacin (see page 140). Interactions can also occur with the antibiotic erythromycin and the heart drug pronestyl.

Probucol

Probucol (Lorelco) is a cholesterol-lowering drug that is chemically unlike any other drug I've discussed. It was one of the earliest drugs developed for this purpose, and while it was a dramatic step forward at the time, it has been largely displaced since then by other medications. Probucol seems to inhibit the oxidation of LDL cholesterol, but the exact mechanism is unknown. At the usual dosage of 1 gram per day, this results in a reduction in total cholesterol of from 10 to 15 percent. Unfortunately, probucol also reduces HDL cholesterol levels, sometimes to a significant degree. It does not affect triglyceride levels at all.

Probucol can have side effects, including flatulence, nausea and vomiting, abdominal pain, and diarrhea. Changes in heart rhythms have been reported, too. Some people also seem to be hypersensitive to the drug's effects. This has produced adverse reactions ranging in severity from rashes to anorexia and impotence in these sensitive individuals.

OTHER MEDICINES TO BE CONCERNED ABOUT

You should be aware that some other prescription medicines can have a negative impact on your cholesterol levels. Progesterones are used in hormone replacement therapy for menopausal women, and are used in birth control pills. Progesterones, especially those that do not contain estrogens, the main female hormones, have been shown to boost LDL cholesterol levels while reducing HDL cholesterol levels by 5 to 15 percent. Anabolic steroids, which are sometimes used to combat muscle wasting in AIDS patients and are frequently abused by athletes, can lower HDL levels by 10 to 70 percent. Anyone using these drugs should only do so under the supervision of a physician.

There are also some medications used to treat high blood pressure that can raise total cholesterol levels, including diuretics and beta-blockers. They do this by boosting LDL cholesterol and triglyceride levels while reducing amounts of the helpful HDL cholesterol. While the beta-blockers appear to increase cholesterol levels more than the diuretics, both can cause significant increases in your cholesterol level. You need to be extremely careful with these medications. If you are currently using these drugs, *never* reduce or discontinue the dosage without the consent of your physician regardless of how good you feel. An abrupt change in the medication level can trigger a stroke or heart attack without warning. In this case, the negative impact of these drugs on cholesterol levels must be weighed against the need to control your high blood pressure.

As you can see, modern medicine has developed a number of potent drugs to help control cholesterol levels. These medications can be very effective in certain circumstances, and are clearly called for in treating advanced heart disease or when the body produces excessive amounts of cholesterol on its own. Most of us, however, need to look at both the positive and negative effects of these drugs. Patients and doctors alike need to examine the benefits as well as the side effects in order to decide whether use of these medications is justified.

Fortunately, modern science has also verified the potential of a number of natural products that work with the body to help reduce cholesterol naturally. My goal is to show people how they can maintain a healthy heart and naturally reduce their chances of developing heart disease by changing their lifestyle and harnessing the hidden power of Nature found in natural products. Fiber, garlic, phytosterols, antioxidants, niacin, and a strain of rice food yeast have all been shown to lower cholesterol levels. We'll look at these natural therapies in the next two chapters.

CHAPTER 9

Cholesterol Reduction and the East-West Connection

One of the major medical discoveries of this century has been the understanding of how cholesterol is regulated in cells. For example, the 1985 Nobel Prize was awarded to Michael Brown and Joseph Goldstein for their discovery of the body's cholesterol-control mechanism. This followed the discovery of a plant- and yeast-derived substance that inhibited cholesterol production some years earlier, which led to the entire class of statin drugs that I described in Chapter 8. But before scientists "discovered" this principle, it already existed in the plant world. The drug-company scientists merely developed a process for purifying and concentrating a plant chemical that occurred naturally, eventually making synthetic and semisynthetic versions of the same chemical.

The benefits of these purified medicines come at a price. These drugs are expensive when you calculate the lifetime costs of a medication. Much of this cost is related to research and development, and the expenses involved in testing and documenting all of the drug's side effects. You may pay for this yourself as a consumer, or it may be paid for by an insurance company or a government program, but the cost is there.

In this chapter, we will look at how the human body has adapted to the plants eaten by our early ancestors, and how this has affected the way our bodies process cholesterol. I'll then introduce you to a natural remedy from China that shows great promise as a safe cholesterol fighter.

PLANTS, HUMANS, AND CHOLESTEROL

Cholesterol control is an important part of many different processes within our bodies, and substances in the plant foods we take into our bodies affect cholesterol usage in many ways. Why do plants have these substances? It may be an accident of Nature. For example, we know that lemons and oranges have substances in their rinds that inhibit the creation of cholesterol. These oils (limonene and geraniol) protect citrus fruits from being attacked by fungi. As a byproduct of making fruit juice, we now use these oils to scent household cleaning agents. In their pure forms, though, these chemicals may have the ability to prevent certain forms of cancer.

Then again, the connection between plants and humans may not be an accident at all. Plants have been on this planet for about a billion years. Modern humans have been here for only 50,000 years. That means we have co-existed with plants since the beginning of human life on this planet. Ecologists and geneticists call this process co-evolution. Our genetic information developed in equilibrium with a great diversity of plants, since prehistoric humans ate plants in large amounts. Our bodies are still adapted to this early diet. For example, it has been estimated that early humans ate fruits containing up to 500 milligrams (mg) of vitamin C per day, so there was never a need for our genes to make enzymes for the manufacture of vitamin C. That may be why our bodies cannot make vitamin C to this day.

Similarly, we needed to hold onto fat in our ancient fat-poor, calorie-poor environment. Since cholesterol lipoproteins contain fat, the genes for cholesterol control were set at a level that would hang onto cholesterol, too. That is the essence of the cholesterol thermostat discussed in Chapter 4. Because our ancient diet contained plant-derived foods with natural cholesterol inhibitors, our bodies adapted to the presence of these substances. As a result, the plants acted to naturally reduce the cholesterol synthesis involved in the growth of certain cells, including the growth of cells in atherosclerotic blood vessels or in tumors.

Our modern diets have changed radically from ancient times, yet the change has occurred so quickly in evolutionary terms that our bodies have not had time to adjust to it. As a result, our cholesterol thermostat is still set where it was a long time ago. Today, humans live much longer, so the effects of having high cholesterol levels over many years leads to heart disease and other problems.

Our approach to medicine has changed, too. We no longer have medicine men and women gathering plants with special medicinal value. Instead, we extract and purify what we call the active principle from natural products to make highly potent drugs (see Chapter 8), and use these as models to design even more potent drugs. In certain situations, these drugs can save lives. However, they can also be overused, which results in as much harm as good. They can also be very expensive.

Antibiotics provide a good example. Antibiotics have been developed to fight infections. If you had a life-threatening infection you would want to have one of these drugs regardless of the expense, because a modern-day antibiotic could save your life. In movies from the 1940s, the football hero would be hospitalized with a fracture received on the game-ending heroic play and would die in the hospital. It was perfectly believable at that time for someone to die of a simple infection resulting from a fracture. Today, you would sue everyone from the hospital director to the corporation that owned the hospital if that happened. This change has come about through the development of antibiotics.

On the other hand, if you have a common cold and your doctor gives you the latest broad-spectrum antibiotic for a viral infection, you receive no benefit—only the side effects. You may experience gastrointestinal upset as the beneficial bacteria in your large intestines are disturbed by the antibiotic. You may also stimulate the growth of resistant bacteria by adding the antibiotic to the mix of the normal bacteria we all have in our bodies.

Recent studies on some cholesterol-lowering drugs have shown that these drugs can prevent heart disease. The drugs can also benefit patients who already have heart disease, including those who have had heart surgery. These valuable studies are among the most exciting developments ever to occur in cardiology. However, in my view, these drugs are not appropriate for heart disease prevention in the general population for two reasons: cost and side effects. The side effects of these drugs, which can include changes in liver function and a rare muscle disease, may be tolerable for patients with advanced heart disease. But to extend the use of these pharmaceuticals to the 25 percent of the population in the United States with high cholesterol levels would be a real problem.

We live in equilibrium with the fungi, yeast, and bacteria on this planet. These living organisms are affected by what we put into our bodies and how we live. Most of the prevention of infection around the world has come about through improved nutrition and sanitation, not through antibiotics. In the same way, I feel that the prevention of chronic diseases will come from natural measures, not drugs with significant side effects. To cite a few examples, I predict we will one day have natural hormone replacement for postmenopausal women, natural contraceptives, and many natural products that will fight the processes involved in cancer, aging, and heart disease.

Scientists are now rediscovering natural products that are able to mimic the actions of the prescription medicines we have been using for years. Researchers are also finding other effects that had been lost when the natural substances were purified to produce the modern cholesterol-lowering drugs. Our challenge is to reintroduce the natural remedies themselves into our diets. This, along with appropriate diet, exercise, and stress reduction, will permit the natural prevention of heart disease.

GOOD NEWS FROM CHINA: A BETTER WAY TO LOWER CHOLESTEROL LEVELS

Herbs have been used in traditional Chinese medicine for thousands of years. Many of these herbs came to China from the Middle East. We know that in the Tigris-Euphrates Valley, the cradle of human civilization, humans used plants with medicinal value for hundreds of generations.

One example of a naturally occurring medicinal substance is a Chinese medicine derived from a yeast called *Monascus purpureus*. This yeast, known to the Chinese as *Hong qu* (pronounced "hong tchew"), was produced using rice in a carefully controlled fermenting process. The Chinese first recorded the medical uses of this natural product for heart conditions during the Ming dynasty (1368–1644). A medical book called the *Ben Cao Gang Mu*, which was written at that time, noted Hong qu's value in the improvement of blood circulation and the reduction of blood clotting. It was also recommended for indigestion and diarrhea, and was said to promote the health of the stomach and spleen. It was noted long ago in China that foods prepared with Hong qu resisted spoilage. That was probably due partly to the cholesterol-inhibiting substances in the yeast. There are also red pigments in the yeast that have antibacterial effects. This also accounts, in part, for the ability of the red coating on Chinese meats to protect against spoilage.

The *Ben Cao Gang Mu*, which is still in print, describes Hong qu as slightly sweet with a mild taste that is very distinctive. (I agree, because I've eaten it myself.) It is used as a food preservative and colorant. The red color of those Peking ducks you sometimes see hanging in Chinese restaurants is due to the pigment in Hong qu.

These pigment extracts do not necessarily have the medically active ingredient, however. Only certain strains of Hong qu have significant amounts of the naturally occurring cholesterol inhibitors. If the wrong strain is used, or if the food yeast is prepared using the wrong fermentation methods, it will not contain optimum levels of all the cholesterol-inhibiting substances in the yeast.

In modern times, we know about the connection between high cholesterol levels and an increased risk of heart disease. Therefore, scientists in both China and the United States have used Hong qu as the basis of cholesterol-lowering dietary supplements. In China, two yeast preparations are used: Xuezhikang ("blood lipid healthy") and Zhitai ("lipid healthy").

Zhitai is a red yeast product that is produced by simply grinding the yeast after the rice is fermented. It is closely related to Hong qu, which is the basis of an American dietary supplement called Cholestin-3. Cholestin-3 is rice and yeast, and is mostly rice by weight (about 99 percent). Xuezhikang is an extract of the Chinese food yeast that is made by mixing the yeast with alcohol and processing it to remove most of the rice gluten. As shown in Chinese studies, Xuezhikang delivers about 40 percent more cholesterol-lowering substances than Cholestin-3 or Zhitai.

It is important to remember that Cholestin-3 is a dietary supplement, not a drug. As such, it is regulated as a food by the Dietary Supplement Health and Education Act, and can thus be sold over the counter to help consumers maintain healthy cholesterol levels. This assumes, of course, that Cholestin-3 is used as part of a heart-healthy lifestyle, which includes proper diet, exercise, and stress reduction (see Chapters 5 through 7). Cholestin-3 has not yet been tested in this country to the extent that Xuezhikang and Zhitai have been tested in China. However, it is not unreasonable to expect results with Cholestin-3 similar to those that have been obtained with the Chinese extracts.

Xuezhikang has undergone significant animal testing, and has been shown to be safe and effective. There was no observed toxicity in rats when Xuezhikang was given as a single dose that was 533 times the usual amount. Then, the rats were given from 33 to 66 times the human dose of Xuezhikang over a four-month period. Their cholesterol levels fell, but there were no changes in liver function, and all their other blood tests were normal. Xuezhikang was also tested in rabbits and quail fed a special diet designed to raise cholesterol levels. Again, the extract lowered both cholesterol and triglyceride levels.

I have reviewed seventeen papers from the Chinese medical literature on human studies done with Xuezhikang and Zhitai. In the studies I reviewed, a total of 872 patients were treated with Xuezhikang or Zhitai. After eight weeks of treatment, total cholesterol levels were reduced by an average of from 28 to 68 milligrams per deciliter (mg/dL), or from 11.2 to 32.2 percent. In eight of these studies there was a comparison to a control group of patients who did not receive the test substances, while in nine studies there were no controls.

One of the most revealing studies was performed at four hospitals in the greater Beijing area. A total of 446 persons participated in this eight-week study. They included 324 individuals who received Xuezhikang and 122 who used another traditional Chinese medicine for high cholesterol levels as a quasi-control group for comparison. Xuezhikang was clearly better than the comparison medicine. Compared with their baseline condition before the experiment began, the group using Xuezhikang had a 23 percent reduction in total serum (blood) cholesterol. This group also experienced a 36.5 percent drop in triglyceride levels, while the concentration of LDL cholesterol declined by 28.5 percent. Meanwhile, HDL cholesterol levels rose by 19.6 percent. (For an explanation of the different types of cholesterol, see Chapter 4.)

These changes in cholesterol levels produced sizable short-term improvements in the cardiovascular health of the study participants. In fact, this natural treatment lowered the value of an index used to predict the probability of atherosclerosis by 34.2 percent.

Another large Chinese study confirmed these results. This study was conducted by Beijing Hospital in 1994. It divided a total of 152 patients into two groups. One group of 101 participants received Zhitai, while 51 others were given a different traditional medicine. All of the patients had high cholesterol levels (more than 250 mg/dL). In eight weeks, Zhitai lowered the average total cholesterol count by 19.2 percent, compared with a 1.5 percent reduction in the control group. Triglyceride levels decreased by 32.1 percent, while LDL levels dropped by 27.4 percent. The amount of good HDL cholesterol jumped by 19.3 percent. The study's authors also observed that the greatest improvements in cholesterol profiles were found in patients who had high total cholesterol and LDL levels, and low HDL levels, to start with.

Despite the dramatic changes that were seen, this natural therapy appears to be quite safe. Less than 1 percent of the participants in these studies had to stop taking the product because of side effects. Minor discomfort was reported in only 3 percent of users. These occasional side effects included acid indigestion and stomach discomfort. There were no observed changes in blood or urine, and no significant impact on liver function.

I believe this natural product can work together with diet and lifestyle changes to lower your cholesterol significantly. Cholestin-3 is now being sold in drug and discount stores throughout the United States. As with almost any drug or natural product, women who are pregnant or nursing should *not* take Cholestin-3. Its safety when used with other medications has not been studied, and you should consult with your doctor if you take blood-thinning medicines, or if you have heart disease, liver disease or other liver condition, or another serious illness.

It has been estimated that 25 percent of the patients who take cholesterol-lowering prescription drugs and follow a low-fat, low-cholesterol diet do not achieve adequate reduction in their cholesterol levels. In many patients, this is due to the presence of elevated triglyceride levels, so physicians must add a second or third drug to lower triglycerides as well. There is some indication from the Chinese studies I have reviewed that Cholestin-3 may lower triglyceride levels. The mechanism for this effect is not known, but may be due to unsaturated fatty acids found in the yeast.

My colleagues and I are repeating these studies under tightly controlled conditions. We are giving Cholestin-3 to American men and women, ages fifty to seventy-five, with both increased and borderline high cholesterol levels in order to see if the product can lower both cholesterol and triglyceride levels. We are using the same procedures to test Cholestin-3 that have been used to test the cholesterol-lowering drugs. This includes use of a placebo, which is an inert substance given to some study participants as a control substance. In addition, neither the patients themselves nor my staff are aware of which patients are getting the placebo and which are getting the Cholestin-3. This is called a double-blind study, and it prevents anyone involved in the study from being swayed by knowledge of who is receiving the substance being tested.

We are also keeping a close eye on the participants' diets during the trial. One study of patients on cholesterol-lowering drugs who signed up for the Pritikin diet program demonstrates that diet and exercise can lead to additional improvements even when prescription drug use is held constant. These individuals had high levels of triglycerides and cholesterol just as the Chinese test subjects did, so it may be that Cholestin-3 works with diet to help lower triglycerides.

How low should your cholesterol level be? As low as you can get it naturally. If you have heart disease, *always* consult your cardiologist before taking any substance. Cholestin-3 is a natural dietary supplement meant to maintain normal heart function in the general population. It is not intended to treat heart disease. However, lowering your cholesterol level can help keep your heart disease from getting worse.

Every day, cardiologists are discovering new treatments for patients with severe heart disease. These new treatments are not an argument against prevention. On the contrary, both are needed. I believe that prevention can be both highly technical and natural by combining a scientific understanding of what is going on in each patient with the use of natural therapies. Just because I favor a natural approach for prevention does not mean that I am opposed to using the best science we have for those who are very sick. As a society, we have to decide what we plan to do with our vast resources. Are our health-care dollars so limited that we can't take care of the very sick and spend money on prevention, too? I don't think so. I believe we can do both. And by organizing our health-care system well, we can pay for both.

The prevention of heart disease through changes in diet, exercise habits, and lifestyle, and through the use of natural products such as Cholestin-3, will ultimately reduce the amount of money we have to spend on bypass operations and other expensive procedures. While new scientific developments in microsurgery will one day make bypass surgery easier on the patient, I still believe that the greatest advances in longevity and quality of life will come from natural therapies and prevention. Natural products such as Cholestin 3 and the products discussed in the next chapter may be an important beginning in the realization of this promise.

CHAPTER 10

Other Natural Medicines

The modern application of natural medicine is in its beginning stages. In ancient times, medicine women and men would collect medicinal plants in the form of cuttings, roots, or berries. These plants were used as part of the food supply or as special medicines to fight disease. Today, we classify natural medicines as dietary supplements to differentiate them from prescription drugs. Prescription drugs are used to treat or prevent specific diseases, while dietary supplements are taken to maintain and promote health, such as maintaining healthy cholesterol levels.

In our day, we have rediscovered several natural medicines, discussed in this chapter, that can help maintain healthy cholesterol levels in a number of ways. *Fiber* traps cholesterol in the intestine and takes it out of the body. *Phytosterols* also work in the intestine by competing with dietary cholesterol for absorption through the intestinal wall. *Soy protein* lowers cholesterol when eaten in place of animal proteins. *Garlic* and *niacin* work within the blood and liver to lower cholesterol production.

Fish oil acts on the circulatory and immune systems. *Aspirin* makes the blood less likely to clot, and thus less likely to form blood-vessel blockages. *Antioxidants*, such as beta-carotene, vitamin C, and vitamin E, may work to slow the process of atherosclerosis. And in some individuals, *B vitamins* can help reduce the risk of heart disease by affecting circulating levels of an amino acid called homocysteine.

Because these various substances work in different ways, you can achieve optimal heart disease prevention by using several of them at once, especially in conjunction with Cholestin-3 (see Chapter 9). This is unlike the use of a single drug for disease prevention. Such a regimen can be as simple or complex as you want. However, remember that these strategies should be combined with changes in your diet and lifestyle (see Chapters 5 through 7). If you have a pre-existing medical condition, you should *always* talk to your doctor before taking supplements of any kind. Now, let's examine each substance.

FIBER: THE CHOLESTEROL TRAPPER

By now, I'm sure you've heard about the benefits of fiber. There has been a great deal of publicity on how fiber can lower cholesterol levels, and how it can reduce the incidence of colon cancer and other diseases. You may not know, however, that not all fiber is created equal. There are two main types of fiber: *water-soluble* and *insoluble*. Water-soluble fibers are gels that can absorb other substances, including the bile acids found in the intestines. This allows water-based fiber to function much like the bile-acid sequestrant drugs discussed in Chapter 8. Insoluble fiber, on the other hand, cannot absorb much of anything. While it is very valuable for its ability to increase bowel regularity, it does not influence cholesterol levels in any way.

Water-soluble fiber dissolves in your intestines but is not absorbed into the bloodstream. Once it dissolves, soluble fiber is able to bind to the cholesterol-based bile acids that are secreted by the liver. The fiber carries these bile acids out of the body. The liver then makes bile acids in an effort to restore the lost acids by drawing cholesterol from the bloodstream. The end result is a lower level of cholesterol in the blood.

Examples of water-soluble fiber include pectins, certain gums, and psyllium. Pectins are found in many fruits in small amounts, so there actually is some truth to the old adage, "An apple a day keeps the doctor away." Pectin supplements are also available. Gums are found in oats and legumes. Oat bran, for example, is higher in gum content than oatmeal, which is why it is more effective in lowering cholesterol levels. Guar gum, extracted from the cluster bean, has been shown to significantly reduce total cholesterol levels. It's also very effective as a thickening agent. Guar gum is frequently added to nonfat versions of foods to replace the sticky fats that these foods normally contain. Unfortunately, you need to eat a great deal of guar gum for it to work. Another good source of gum is the legume family of vegetables. Excellent choices include pinto, lima, red, and navy beans, as well as lentils and split peas. However, keep in mind that while beans will add fiber to your diet, they will also add calories. Thus, you should limit your intake of beans.

Psyllium is derived from the seed husks of a plant that originally grew in India. It is contained in Metamucil and several other commercial fiber supplements, and is sometimes added to cereals. Psyllium is a source of soluble and insoluble fiber, and has been shown to lower cholesterol levels when used several times a day.

For maximum effect, you should take psyllium with your meals. This will also improve your regularity.

Several studies have shown that soluble fiber is effective in reducing the amount of cholesterol and other lipids in the blood. A study conducted at the University of Kentucky Medical School by Dr. James Anderson showed a significant drop in total cholesterol when soluble fiber was added to the diets of 146 people with moderately elevated cholesterol levels. The study participants were divided into three groups. The first group continued eating their usual diets, while the second group ate a low-fat diet that included 15 grams, or more than half an ounce, of fiber a day. The third group followed a low-fat diet that contained 25 grams of fiber. This fiber came from ordinary foods, such as oatmeal or canned beans. After a year, the first group showed a drop of 7 percent in their total cholesterol levels, even though they supposedly maintained a constant diet. This reduction may have been due to small changes the people in this group made because they knew they were being studied. The group that ate 15 grams of fiber had a 9 percent drop in their total cholesterol levels, while the group that ate 25 grams showed a decline of 13 percent.

Two studies at the Stanford University School of Medicine showed that soluble fiber reduces levels of LDL cholesterol. The doctors who conducted the first study gave 15 grams of soluble fiber per day to sixteen people. The fiber was in the form of a pectin and psyllium supplement. After one month, LDL levels dropped an average of 12.4 percent. Total cholesterol fell by 8.3 percent. The second study found a correlation between LDL levels and the amount of soluble fiber consumed. Persons who ate 5 grams of soluble fiber daily for a month showed a reduction in LDL levels of 5.6 percent, while those who consumed 15 grams experienced a decline of 14.9 percent. (For an explanation of the different types of cholesterol, see Chapter 4.)

Insoluble fiber is less digestible than water-soluble fiber. It largely passes unchanged through the intestine and is eliminated in the stool. Much of the insoluble fiber we eat is cellulose, a carbohydrate that provides much of the physical structure of plants. It is found in prodigious amounts in wheat bran, celery, and many other natural, unprocessed foods. Because insoluble fiber is poorly digested, its primary role is to add bulk to the stool. This helps increase regularity, while adding enough roughage to help clean off the walls of the intestine as the waste products move along. These two qualities improve the functioning of the large intestine, so much so that studies have shown a correlation between the intake of insoluble fiber and the incidence of colon cancer. Unfortunately, the inability to trap bile acids keeps this type of fiber from being effective in lowering cholesterol levels. While you should continue to eat insoluble fiber for its many other health benefits, it will not reduce your cholesterol level.

Some people experience gastrointestinal distress when they start taking large amounts of fiber. This problem usually goes away, however, as the intestines adjust to healthier levels of fiber. In order to minimize the gas or bloating that may occur, be sure to add fiber to your diet slowly. Also, spread out your fiber consumption. You don't want to eat all of your fiber at one sitting, since that could be too big of a jolt for your body. It's better to eat high-fiber foods at each meal. You should drink plenty of water, too. This will give the soluble fiber all of the water it needs to perform its cholesterol-lowering function, and will keep you from becoming constipated.

The best way to get more fiber into your diet is to eat a combination of beans and other legumes, high-fiber cereals and grains, and high-fiber fruits and vegetables. These foods also provide you with other advantages, such as natural antioxidants and additional nutrients.

There are some traps to watch out for. Many breads use bleached "enriched" flour. Use of this flour denies you the fiber and other natural products found in whole grains. For example, high-fiber rye bread is heavier and less airy than enriched-flour rye. Beans are a good source of fiber, but if you are watching your weight you have to watch out for the calories beans contain. For example, I found a recipe for a bean soup in a famous nutritionist's book that provided more than 500 calories a serving. To avoid these and other pitfalls, carefully read the labels on the foods you buy.

Table 10.1 will give you some guidelines that may help you increase your fiber intake to more than 25 grams a day. Remember, soluble fiber is important for its ability to remove cholesterol from the body, while a high total fiber count may help prevent colon cancer and other digestive problems. It's also important to *not* increase your total calorie count.

Table 10.1. Higher-Fiber Foods and Supplements

Choose ...	Fiber (gm)	Soluble Fiber (gm)	Rather than ...	Soluble Fiber (gm)	Fiber (gm)
Cereals					
Oatmeal	9.5	4.9	Cream of Wheat	3.8	1.6
Cheerios	9.1	4.2	Rice Krispies	1.2	0.3
Bran Buds	36.0	10.0	Shredded Wheat	12.5	1.6
All Bran	30.8	5.1	Raisin Bran	13.5	2.4
Beans					
Black beans	7.1	2.8	Black-eyed peas	3.9	0.4
Pinto beans	6.2	2.2	Cooked split peas	3.2	1.1
Butter beans	7.3	2.9	Cooked chickpeas	5.3	1.6

Choose . . .	Fiber (gm)	Soluble Fiber (gm)	Rather than . . .	Soluble Fiber (gm)	Fiber (gm)
Fruits					
Figs (dried)	8.2	4.0	Fruit juices without pulp		
Pears	3.5	1.3			
Apples	2.0	0.6			
Oranges	2.0	1.0			
Bananas	1.9	0.6			
Raisins	2.3	1.1			
Vegetables					
Brussels sprouts	5.7	3.0	Asparagus	2.0	0.8
Broccoli	3.1	1.5	Corn	2.9	0.5
Carrots	3.2	1.5	Cooked spinach	1.8	0.6
Sweet potatoes	2.5	1.1	White potatoes	2.0	1.0
Fiber Supplements					
Citrus pectin (1 tbsp)	5.5	5.5	Citrucel (1 tbsp)	2.0	2.0
Profibe (1 scoop)	5.0	5.0	Flax fiber (2 tbsp)	5.7	2.2
Sugar Free Metamucil (1 tbsp)	6.0	5.2	Metamucil (1 tbsp)	5.4	4.2

All fiber contents are based on a 3.5-ounce portion. The number of calories differ from item to item, and you need to take this into consideration. For more complete information, consult *Fat & Fiber* by Art Ulene (Avery Publishing Group).

PHYTOSTEROLS: THE CHOLESTEROL COMPETITORS

As their name implies, phytosterols ("sterols" for short) are plant substances chemically related to cholesterol. There are more than fifty phytosterols in Nature. Some are only found in particular plant species, while others are prevalent throughout the plant kingdom. By far, the most widespread is *sitosterol*, technically known as beta sitosterol. Two other sterols are *campesterol* and *stigmasterol*.

Phytosterols perform a variety of essential functions in plants and animals. Ergosterol, for example, is considered to be the nucleus of dietary vitamin D, which is an important source for this vitamin along with the vitamin D created when your skin is exposed to sunlight. The fortification of foods with vitamin D led to the disappearance of rickets, a disease common in industrial-age England, where there was little sunlight and few dietary sources of vitamin D.

Sitosterol is almost chemically identical to cholesterol. This similarity helps sitosterol, and to a lesser extent all phytosterols, to perform their various functions. Phytosterols compete with dietary cholesterol for absorption through the small intestine, which reduces the amount of cholesterol that gets into your bloodstream. Sterols do not affect the cholesterol thermostat, the cholesterol-control mechanism described in Chapter 4.

Phytosterols are found in an assortment of food products. Legumes are an excellent source, especially peas and kidney beans. Wheat germ is also high in sterols. Fruits and nonlegume vegetables have phytosterols in relatively small amounts. Oranges are best among the fruits, followed by bananas. Apples, cherries, peaches, and pears have anywhere from a half to a third of the phytosterol content found in oranges. Beets and Brussels sprouts are your best choices in vegetables, followed by cauliflower. Vegetables with lower sterol concentrations include cabbage, carrots, onions, and yams. Phytosterols are also found in nuts and vegetable oils, but you should stay away from these foods to reduce your fat intake.

A number of nutritional supplement companies are now making sitosterol products that can be purchased at most health, drug, and discount stores. Sitosterol supplements are effective only when you use them correctly. But remember that the phytosterols work by binding onto cholesterol in the intestine. In order to keep this cholesterol from being assimilated, the plant sterols need to be mixed in with your food as it moves down the intestinal passage. So, for optimal results, consume your phytosterols with your meals. This increases the likelihood that they will be able to latch onto the cholesterol. Consuming them before or after your meal will reduce their efficacy, because the phytosterols will be either ahead of or behind the food as it makes its way to your large intestine.

As with prescription drugs, you need to take phytosterols every day. When phytosterol use is stopped, your cholesterol levels will rise within several weeks. Sitosterol and the other phytosterols are so similar to cholesterol that the body does not react negatively to them. Also, sitosterol does not lose its effectiveness when taken over a period of time. However, if you eat very low levels of dietary cholesterol, you will see little or no effect on your cholesterol levels when using sitosterol.

SOY PROTEIN: THE MEAT SUBSTITUTE THAT LOWERS CHOLESTEROL LEVELS

Soy protein has been revered for its life-giving properties as a food and as a medicine since ancient times. The soybean, which came to China via camel caravans from the Middle East, was one of the sacred crops of the Chinese emperor Sheng-nung. In 800 A.D., soy protein made its way to Japan, and was brought to Europe in the seventeenth century. Soybeans came to the United States by accident, as ballast in ships crossing the Atlantic.

What makes soy protein different from other vegetable proteins? All proteins are made of building blocks called amino acids. Most vegetables do not contain all the amino acids the body requires. That's why vegetarians mix beans, lentils, or peas with rice or corn to get complete proteins at each meal. One the other hand, soybeans provide an almost perfect set of amino acids.

In Asia, soy is eaten as tofu, tempeh, miso soup, and other forms. There, the average daily intake of soy protein is between 40 and 100 grams. In the United States, it is less than 5 grams a day.

In an analysis of twenty-nine clinical studies on soy protein, Dr. Anderson of the University of Kentucky concluded that the substitution of soy protein for animal protein led to lower cholesterol levels, although no one knows how this occurs. The daily consumption in these studies was between 31 grams and 47 grams a day. Since soy also contains antioxidants called isoflavones, it may help prevent heart disease in ways other than by simply lowering cholesterol levels.

If you have a high cholesterol level, you can add thirty grams of soy protein to your daily meals by drinking two glasses of soy milk (4 to 10 grams each) and eating a serving of a soy-based meat substitute (18 grams). You can also buy a soy protein powder containing Supro or Purasoy, which has twenty grams in two scoops. Thus, two drinks per day made with two scoops each will give you 40 grams a day. Using soy powder also lets you receive a measured amount of isoflavones a day. I believe that foods bioengineered to contain soy protein will eventually play a major role in disease prevention.

GARLIC: THE OVERALL HEART HELPER

Garlic, known botanically as *Allium sativum*, is grown throughout the world. It was one of humankind's earliest medical discoveries. Sanskrit records dating back more than five thousand years note the medicinal benefits of garlic. The Greek physician Hippocrates also wrote about the herb's many uses, as did the Chinese. Folk tales and ancient records from around the world attest to garlic's long-standing use as an antifungal, antiviral, and antibacterial agent. Traditional societies have used garlic to treat everything from dandruff to fevers to swelling. The Bedouins in Arabic countries even use garlic combined with saliva as a very effective antidote for the poison in scorpion stings.

When garlic is crushed, it releases a pungent oil, allicin, that is then converted into several sulfur-bearing compounds responsible for most of garlic's multiple benefits, including the lowering of cholesterol and triglyceride levels. Allicin also boosts the levels of two blood enzymes with antioxidant properties, catalase and glutathione peroxidase. These antioxidants help your body neutralize free radicals. Free radicals are molecules that can lead to the oxidation, or rancidity, of cholesterol and hasten the atherosclerotic process. (See Chapter 4 and page 146.)

A wide variety of studies have confirmed garlic's ancient role as a natural medicine. Researchers have learned that garlic inhibits the clumping of blood cells called platelets, which makes the blood less sticky and reduces the blood's tendency to clot. This, in turn, reduces the risk of an artery becoming obstructed by a blood clot.

A number of studies have shown that garlic has a beneficial effect on the blood, including a modest ability to reduce cholesterol levels and blood pressure. But in order to get these benefits, you need to consume a lot of garlic. While adding a clove to your meal will enhance its flavor, it will have just a modest effect on the fats in your bloodstream. The studies showed statistically significant changes only when the daily dosage was between 600 mg and 900 mg of standardized garlic extract per day. Although you could eat enough raw garlic to get the equivalent therapeutic dosage, the resulting odor on your breath would make your treatment procedure obvious to everyone (not all of whom would be sympathetic). A better option is to use odor-reduced garlic tablets. (There is no such thing as active odor-free garlic, since it is the allicin that smells.) These tablets are widely available at health, drug, and discount stores, and are far more convenient than constantly crushing raw garlic. Start off with one 500 mg tablet per day and then boost the dosage to between two to four tablets per day after a week or two. Garlic's power to improve the health of your blood will give you a major boost in your efforts to lower your cholesterol levels.

NIACIN: THE ALL-AROUND CHOLESTEROL FIGHTER

You have no doubt heard of niacin as one of the B vitamins. Back in 1917, scientists discovered that the substance we now know as niacin could prevent pellagra, a condition characterized by gastrointestinal disturbances and skin inflammations, as well as various nervous and mental disorders. Twenty years later, researchers at the University of Wisconsin isolated niacin as a nutrient.

Niacin is used by the liver to form niacinamide, a compound that is sometimes used instead of niacin as the ingredient in multivitamin tablets. The use of niacinamide as a supplement appears to be perfectly acceptable for the prevention of pellegra. However, it makes a big difference exactly which substance is used when it comes to lowering your cholesterol levels. While niacin has been shown to be very effective in reducing cholesterol levels, niacinamide has no effect on cholesterol levels whatsoever.

It appears that niacin reduces cholesterol levels during its conversion to niacinamide in the liver. So if you provide your body with niacinamide to start with, no conversion is necessary, and there is no improvement in your cholesterol levels. This is not a big concern as far as multivitamin tablets are concerned, since the amount of niacin or niacinamide provided is usually quite low. However, if you are taking large dosages of niacin in order to lower your cholesterol levels, it is vitally important that you only use niacin and *not* niacinamide.

Niacin reduces cholesterol through several different mechanisms. As I noted in Chapter 4, most of your body's cholesterol is manufactured inside your liver. While scientists aren't sure exactly how this happens, they do know that as niacin is converted to niacinamide several changes occur. Niacin decreases the liver's production of VLDL, which carries both triglycerides and cholesterol throughout the body. The higher the concentration of VLDL and LDL in the bloodstream, the more likely it is that atherosclerotic plaque will develop, since VLDL is converted to LDL and promotes atherosclerosis itself. So niacin's ability to lower VLDL production may help reduce the buildup of plaque.

Niacin stimulates the formation of prostaglandins. These chemicals are involved in a wide variety of body functions, including the maintenance of healthy blood vessels. Niacin is also able to boost the production of a blood chemical called PGI2, which is involved in platelet clumping. The more PGI2 you have, the less likely your blood is to clot. This reduces the likelihood that you will develop a potentially fatal blood clot. Niacin's stimulation of PGI2 also helps to thin the blood and slow down the process of atherosclerosis.

Yet another benefit of niacin is its ability to lower triglyceride levels in the blood. It does this by increasing the activity level of lipoprotein lipase, a chemical that pushes more of the triglycerides in the VLDL out of the bloodstream and into the tissues. The correlation between lower triglyceride levels in the bloodstream and a reduced incidence of cardiovascular disease provides yet another reason to supplement your diet with niacin.

There is a large number of studies on niacin. While much of this research has examined niacin in combination with prescription drugs, several studies have confirmed niacin's benefits when taken by itself. One report from the University of Minnesota Medical School noted that most studies show reductions in LDL levels of between 20 and 30 percent, with increases in protective HDL levels of about 20 percent. This is equal to a boost in HDL concentrations of from 10 to 15 milligrams a deciliter (mg/dL). These benefits, which are comparable to the results achieved by drugs such as gemfibrozil (Lopid) and cholestyramine (Questran), were achieved with dosages of between 3 to 6 grams of niacin per day, which should only be taken while under a physician's care.

An Italian study published in the *American Journal of Cardiology* showed a 20 percent rise in HDL levels when niacin was used. The scientists also reported a 15 to 20 percent drop in total cholesterol and a 45 to 50 percent reduction in triglycerides. Dosages were similar to the dosages used in the Minnesota study.

Niacin has even been shown to reduce mortality rates. A study of men who survived their first heart attack was begun in 1966. Half the study participants received niacin, while the other half were given a placebo. After fifteen years, the niacin group had sixty-nine fewer deaths, which represented an 11 percent drop in mortality compared with the control group. The niacin group lived an average of 1.63 years longer than the placebo group. Another study called the Coronary Drug Project showed that niacin lowers the rate of nonfatal heart attacks by 29 percent.

Niacin tablets come in a variety of sizes, ranging from 50 mg to 750 mg. For best results, you should use a timed-release formula such as Slo-Niacin. This slows the assimilation of the niacin over a period of several hours, which keeps the liver from getting excessive amounts of niacin at any one time. This assures a more constant reduction in VLDL production. Other benefits of niacin use, including the boosts in HDL and PGI2 levels, are also more consistent when timed-release formulas are used. When you begin taking niacin, you should start with a low dose. I usually start patients at 100 mg three times per day, and then increase the dosage by half every week until they are taking 1,000 mg a day. For most people, the maximum dosage ever needed is 1,500 milligrams per day.

I also recommend that you take niacin with your meals to avoid any gastrointestinal upset. Of course, it's always best to eat low-fat, low-cholesterol meals with high levels of fiber-rich fruits and vegetables. That way you can keep the amount of dietary cholesterol that enters your bloodstream to a minimum, allowing the niacin to be used mainly for controlling your body's own cholesterol production.

Niacin can often have minor side effects, particularly when you start taking it. While these side effects are rarely serious, they can cause distress to the uninitiated. Many people experience a flush at the beginning of their niacin use. This totally harmless flush can cause a tingly sensation on the skin, usually on the chest, arms, shoulders, and back. The skin may turn pink or even red, just as it would from blushing or a sunburn. Scientists feel the flush has something to do with the release of the prostaglandins I mentioned earlier, although they can't completely explain why it happens. What they do know is that the effect is strictly limited to your skin, so there's no cause for concern. Taking half an aspirin tablet with the niacin seems to reduce the flushing significantly. The timed-release brands of niacin cause less flushing than the immediate-release versions. With continued niacin use, the amount of flushing usually declines, so it tends to be a temporary problem.

Other, less frequent side effects include gastric upset and rash. Unlike a flush, the rash does not go away within a few minutes. It can continue for several days after you stop taking niacin. Fortunately, these rashes are quite rare. Blurred vision is another infrequent side effect, but it too disappears after the niacin is discontinued. For people whose livers have been damaged by disease or alcohol abuse, niacin can also cause nausea and vomiting. Because of the potential complications, persons with liver disease, peptic ulcers, diabetes, gout, or severe heart arrhythmias should *never* take large dosages of niacin.

Because of the potential side effects, you should consult with your physician before beginning niacin use. As I indicated, these negative consequences are extremely rare, but that's small consolation if you're the one affected by them. The frequency of these side effects is also much less than that encountered with prescription drugs, so you need to keep things in perspective. Niacin is much less expensive than these drugs too, which your pocketbook will certainly appreciate. Just take it easy in the beginning, and slowly build up to your full niacin dosage. That will minimize any problems you might have. For nearly everyone, niacin can be a very valuable weapon in the fight against high cholesterol levels.

FISH OIL: THE "GOOD FAT"

The body fat of cold-water fish such as herring and tuna is rich in fats called fish oils. These oils are rich in substances called *omega-3 fatty acids*. Fish get these oils from eating marine algae.

The body contains two classes of fatty acids, the omega-3s and the omega-6s. (The numbers refer to the chemical composition of each class.) Omega-6s are found in most vegetable oils, including those found in many processed foods, as well as in animals who eat feed sources high in omega-6s. Omega-3s are found not only in fish oils and marine algae, but also in flaxseed oil.

Good health depends on maintaining a balance between the two classes of fatty acids, which both perform numerous important functions. However, changes in the modern diet have upset this balance by drastically reducing the amounts of omega-3 fatty acids consumed by most Americans. This lack of balance often results in inflammations of various kinds throughout the body.

The omega-3s in fish oils produce an anti-inflammatory response, and have been reported to successfully decrease arthritis pain in patients with rheumatoid arthritis. Omega-3s also produce a lowering of triglyceride levels, and make platelets less sticky and less likely to form clots. (However, trials using fish oils to stop clotting of vessels after bypass operations have been disappointing.)

Fish oils have a positive effect on cholesterol levels, especially when you consume them as part of a meal that includes fish. A number of studies have shown as much as a 10 percent reduction in cholesterol levels when fish is substituted for red meat in the diet several nights per week. Also, most fish other than salmon, trout, and catfish are low in fat. So eating fish will not only give you the beneficial fish oils, but the reduced level of fat in your diet will independently lower your cholesterol level, too. Fish and flaxseed oils are available in supplement form.

ASPIRIN: THE BLOOD THINNER

Aspirin is a product that originally was derived from the bark of the willow tree. It causes platelets to become less sticky, which makes the blood less likely to clot. This fights one important part of the process leading to heart disease. Unfortunately, the downside of using aspirin is that it slightly increases the risk of dying from a stroke. This is because blood vessels in the brain are more likely to bleed uncontrollably during a stroke if you are taking aspirin. However, if you have known heart disease, or have had a heart bypass operation or angioplasty, then taking aspirin makes sense. Small doses of aspirin (half a tablet per day) work as well as do larger doses in providing this protection. The final decision on whether or not to use aspirin depends on your overall risk factors, so consult with your physician before taking aspirin on a regular basis.

ANTIOXIDANTS: THE RANCIDITY FIGHTERS

As I have mentioned, it is the oxidized form of cholesterol that is most likely to settle in the arterial walls and cause trouble. This oxidation, or rancidity, is caused by molecules called *free radicals*. Free radical production is related to the body's use of oxygen. Most of the oxygen we breathe is expelled as carbon dioxide. However, some of it is converted into water. Most of the time, this conversion happens immediately. Sometimes, though, the process takes a little longer, and the oxygen can assume very unstable forms called free radicals until the process is completed. Free radicals are also formed in the body by tobacco smoke, ultraviolet radiation, and environmental pollution.

These unstable oxygen molecules can react with other molecules around them, which can cause havoc by severely damaging cells. While our bodies have developed a number of defense mechanisms against free radicals, the effectiveness of these mechanisms declines with age.

Free radicals are involved in the development of atherosclerosis in several ways. The process of plaque buildup begins when free radicals injure the wall of the artery, causing a lesion. In an attempt to repair the damage, white-blood cells called monocytes leave the bloodstream and enter the artery wall. Once there, the monocytes are converted into macrophages that eat up fat and cholesterol, particularly LDL that has been oxidized by free radicals. After they are loaded up with LDL, however, the macrophages become stuck in the cell wall and cannot escape. Unfortunately, macrophages also contain several chemical systems that can generate large quantities of free radicals by themselves. This leads to a self-perpetuating cycle, in which the macrophage oxidizes LDL while attracting even more monocytes from the blood to absorb the LDL that it itself released. The end result is a buildup of atherosclerotic plaque. (Also see Chapters 2 and 4.) Free radicals are also involved in other aspects of cardiovascular disease.

Antioxidants are substances that act as scavengers. They circulate throughout the body in search of free radicals, which they neutralize. With fewer free radicals around to cause problems, the body's tissues can go about their normal business for a longer period of time. This may also slow the aging process, since the body may not sustain the cumulative effects of the damage caused by the estimated 7,000 free radical "hits" we endure every day.

Antioxidants that can reach the cholesterol trapped in the blood vessel wall help to retard the process of atherosclerosis. We do not yet know what is the right balance of these antioxidants for optimum health. Some of them dissolve in fat, others in water. These different solubilities may indicate where they act in the body's cells.

Almost all fruits and vegetables have a certain level of antioxidants as a natural defense mechanism. Cholestin-3, for example, has certain red-colored antioxidants that are also found in some Chinese red spices (see Chapter 9). Three of the most popular antioxidants available in supplement form are beta-carotene, vitamin C, and vitamin E.

Beta-carotene is a precursor to vitamin A, which means that the body can manufacture this vitamin from the raw materials in beta-carotene. Unlike vitamin A, which is toxic in high dosages, beta-carotene will not cause a toxicity problem since the conversion of beta-carotene to vitamin A is carefully controlled by the body. Beta-carotene works well in the presence of fats, which aid in its absorption.

Many consumers became concerned about beta-carotene supplementation when two National Cancer Institute studies showed that heavy smokers had an increased incidence of lung cancer when taking beta-carotene over a seven-year period during which they continued to smoke. No such adverse effects were noted in nonsmoking men in the Health Professional Follow-Up Study. However, the study did not show any benefit from beta-carotene for heart disease, either. The proper role of beta-carotene in heart disease prevention has not been established.

Vitamin C (ascorbic acid) is another powerful antioxidant. It is a water-soluble vitamin, which means that the body cannot store it. Vitamin C inactivates free radicals in blood plasma, as well as the fluid between the body's cells, and other water-soluble areas of the body. Equally important, it has the power to restore vitamin E to its original form after that vitamin has been converted to an oxidized form.

A substantial body of evidence shows that vitamin C reduces cardiovascular disease. One famous study was conducted by Dr. James Enstrom at UCLA. He reviewed ten years' worth of survey data. He found that a group of people who took supplemental vitamin C in amounts ranging from five to ten times the Recommended Dietary Allowance (RDA) had a death rate from heart disease, strokes, and other cardiovascular diseases that was 42 percent lower than that of a group of people who did not take vitamin C supplements. (This study also showed that vitamin C reduced the male death rate from cancer by 25 percent, and from diabetes and infectious diseases by about 15 percent.) Other studies have found that vitamin C reduces the levels of LDL while increasing the concentration of HDL.

Vitamin E is a mixture of closely related compounds called tocopherols. It is fat-soluble and is found primarily in cell membranes and lipoproteins. There it neutralizes free radicals by combining with them to form a nonreactive molecule.

Vitamin E is one of the most commonly used antioxidants. More physicians supplement their own diets with vitamin E than with any other dietary supplement. The Health Professional Follow-Up Study of 39,910 men aged forty to seventy-five found that the 20 percent of participants taking the most vitamin E had a 40 percent lower risk of heart disease. This famous study, conducted by the Harvard School of Public Health, demonstrated a benefit at levels of vitamin E intake that could realistically only be achieved by vitamin supplementation. The Scottish Heart Study found that the risk of undiagnosed coronary heart disease was significantly lower in the 20 percent taking the highest amount of vitamin E among 10,359 men and women aged forty to fifty-nine.

Numerous studies have shown that vitamin E reduces the rate of heart disease. In a six-year study, 147 volunteers were assigned to receive either 100 International Units (IU) of vitamin E daily or a placebo. None of the seventy-four individuals taking vitamin E experienced any heart disease, compared with seven individuals with heart disease in the placebo group. Clinical trials are underway in the Women's Health Study and in another prevention trial involving patients with heart disease. These trials will examine the relationship between cardiovascular disease in women and antioxidant supplements including vitamin E.

In order to minimize your risk of atherosclerosis and other cardiovascular diseases, you should include plenty of antioxidants in your diet. While it is always wise to include large portions of the fruits, whole grains, and vegetables that contain these nutrients, you will also need to take antioxidant supplements to get the greatest possible benefit. I recommend the following daily dosages of antioxidants:

- Vitamin C—250 to 500 mg a day
- Vitamin E—200 to 400 IU a day

A combination antioxidant is usually easier to take, but many people also prefer to take vitamin E and C separately.

B VITAMINS AND HOMOCYSTEINE

In normal individuals, there is a natural variation in the circulating levels of an amino acid, or protein building block, called homocysteine. Individuals with levels of homocysteine that are high, but within the normal range, have been found to have an increased incidence of atherosclerosis and premature heart disease. There is also a rare inherited disease called cystathione beta synthase deficiency, or CBS disease. Persons with CBS disease often have an early onset of heart disease as well as high levels of homocysteine in their blood. Some studies have shown that certain B vitamins, including folate, B_6, and B_{12}, lower homocysteine levels in individuals with heart disease and high levels of homocysteine. This presumably reduces their risk of heart disease. You can obtain this benefit from a standard multivitamin/multimineral capsule taken daily.

Vitamin supplements are purified natural medicines. One day, we may develop other natural medicines that combine the effects of these multiple dietary supplements. Until that time, it is probably wise to include a multimineral/multivitamin tablet in your supplement regimen. If you are a man, you should check your iron status to be sure you are not a carrier of the gene for the iron-overload disease called hemochromatosis. If you carry this gene, which is found in one of every 250 men, you should not take iron supplements. High iron levels also act as pro-oxidants. This could theoretically promote atherosclerosis in everyone, so don't go overboard with your iron supplements. One Scandinavian study found an association between high iron intake and increased rates of atherosclerosis in men consuming a high-fat diet. As a result, many experts feel that women over fifty years of age and men of all ages should not take iron with their multivitamins. There is a variety of good multivitamin/multimineral supplements available without iron for this purpose.

I suspect that you are probably feeling overwhelmed with information at this point. Hang in there! In the next chapter I will put all of these approaches together and show you how you can organize your natural remedies for a healthy heart.

CHAPTER 11

Putting It All Together

e've covered a lot of ground so far. We've seen how atherosclerosis develops. We've looked at some of the risk factors for heart disease, and at how the body's cholesterol thermostat can create more cholesterol than we really need. We've discussed how important diet, stress reduction, and exercise are in maintaining a heart-healthy lifestyle. Finally, we've examined some natural therapies that can lower cholesterol levels as effectively as prescription drugs can, but without the side effects.

Now that you have all of this information, it's time to put it to work. Here's a simple way to integrate all this information into a reasonable plan for maintaining a healthy heart.

GET YOUR CHOLESTEROL LEVEL CHECKED

While there is a lot more to heart disease than just a high cholesterol level, it is still important to have your cholesterol level checked. Such checks can identify people who don't have heart disease but who would benefit from natural cholesterol reduction. This type of screening is also important because it raises awareness about the importance of cholesterol as a risk factor, which may lead to a lowering of cholesterol levels in entire communities. By screening early in life, even in childhood, doctors can obtain an idea of any one individual's risk of developing heart disease. Screening can be used as a way to modify lifestyle choices and decrease the risks of heart disease and other diseases while improving one's quality of life.

I recommend that you get your cholesterol checked every five years if you are under the age of forty, and once a year if you are over forty. Be sure to take this test after you have fasted for at least twelve hours. If your cholesterol level is over 200 mg/dL (see Chapter 3), find out as much as you can by getting a breakdown of your LDL and HDL levels and getting your triglyceride level checked. Discuss the results with your physician. Then decide what to do. The natural therapies you have read about in this book, including lifestyle changes and the use of natural products, will allow you to reduce your cholesterol levels and risk of heart disease without the liver and muscle problems associated with cholesterol-lowering drugs.

So, how "high" is high? While governmental agencies have attempted to set a level for high cholesterol, there is no absolute level at which high cholesterol begins. You will hear the number 240 mg/dL as the level at which you should consult a doctor. You will hear that 300 mg/dL is really high. The fact is that cholesterol, like body weight, is simply a marker for what may be occurring within the body. It is not like a disease with a single cause. Therefore, in order to maintain a healthy cholesterol level, you should maintain a healthy weight, and a healthy level of exercise and other stress-reducing behaviors.

REDUCE YOUR RISK FACTORS

Which risk factors apply to you? Is your cholesterol level normal or high? Are you at your ideal weight? Is your triglyceride level elevated? Are you a smoker? Is your blood pressure high? Do you have a family history of heart disease? If the answer to any of these questions is yes, then you must take a focused approach to reduce the risk factor that stands out most. As you learned in Chapter 3, when you change one risk factor you also lessen the impact of other risk factors. For example, if you reduce your blood pressure, you also reduce the impact of high levels of cholesterol in the blood. I won't waste your time discussing smoking as a risk factor. You know that if you smoke you should quit, but what about body weight, cholesterol, triglycerides, and high blood pressure? Here are two examples to help you understand how risk factors interact. Remember that these are only two of a number of different situations.

Situation One: High Cholesterol Level, Normal Triglyceride Level, Normal Blood Pressure, Normal Weight

If this is you, then your main problem is your cholesterol thermostat (see Chapter 4 for an explanation). You should change your diet to take in more fiber by eating more fruits, vegetables, cereals, and grains. A cereal with water-soluble fiber, such as oatmeal, will help. Other natural fibers that lower cholesterol include guar gum and pectin (see Chapter 10). They are found in many food products. If you want to use a fiber supplement, then Metamucil or psyllium seed husk taken three times per day will work. On the other hand, methylcellulose supplements such as Citrucel do not lower cholesterol levels.

Just taking in more fiber won't bring your cholesterol

level down very much, because ultimately your body will begin to make its own cholesterol to replace what the fiber has absorbed. At this point, you should use an HMG-CoA reductase inhibitor to reduce cholesterol production. Until recently, you would have had to choose from a number of statin drugs to accomplish this, but now Cholestin-3 may be able to perform this function for you (see Chapters 8 and 9). What you should see after eight to twelve weeks of Cholestin-3 use is a decrease in blood cholesterol levels. If you are already taking a statin drug, you should consult with your doctor to see whether a trial with Cholestin-3 is worthwhile. If your cholesterol is greater than 240 mg/dL, or if you have a number of other risk factors (see Chapter 3), see your doctor to be sure that dietary supplementation is appropriate. Remember, it takes eight to twelve weeks to see an effect, since cholesterol recirculates via the bile among the gallbladder, liver, and intestines.

The use of Cholestin-3 rather than a statin drug may help you prevent heart disease at a lower cost and with fewer side effects of these drugs. Your other priorities are to exercise regularly, follow the diet I mentioned in Chapter 5, and take a multivitamin/multimineral tablet and antioxidants (see Chapter 10). The multivitamin/ multimineral should have 400 micrograms (mcg) of folic acid to deal with a potential homocysteine metabolism problem. Your daily antioxidant regimen should include at least 200 to 400 IU of vitamin E and 250 to 500 mg of vitamin C. You should also consider cooking with garlic or taking garlic supplements. Niacin, phytosterols, and fish oils may provide you with additional protection.

Situation Two: High Cholesterol Level, High Triglyceride Level, High Blood Pressure, Overweight

What is the single most important risk factor that you

can reduce? It's obesity. Excess body fat can raise blood pressure, and blood levels of triglycerides and cholesterol. A weight loss of as little as twenty pounds can significantly affect your blood pressure and, in some individuals, lower triglyceride and cholesterol levels. So you should first try to lose weight using the dietary principles outlined in Chapter 5 and the exercise principles discussed in Chapter 7. As you lose weight, you will notice that your stress levels will drop as well. Along with this will come a reduction in blood pressure.

Be sure to consult with your doctor or pharmacist when you put this plan into action. As you lose weight, the blood-pressure medicines that you are taking may make your blood pressure drop below normal. This will make you feel tired or faint. If you stop your blood pressure medications, you will feel better. But watch out! If you regain your weight, your blood pressure can rise again. This is why I always favor staying on your blood-pressure medication during the weight-loss phase, in case you have trouble sticking with your diet. On the other hand, I have had many patients who lost weight and never needed their blood-pressure medications again.

Once you have lost weight, you will notice that your triglyceride and cholesterol levels will have dropped. Are they still above desirable levels? You may be one of those people who has inherited the tendency to hang onto body fat and a cholesterol thermostat that is set at too high a level (see Chapter 4). You should consult your doctor or pharmacist about a trial with Cholestin-3 or a statin drug. If you are already taking a statin, talk with your doctor to see whether a trial with Cholestin-3 is warrented. Remember, it takes from eight to twelve weeks to see an effect, since cholesterol recirculates via the bile among the gallbladder, liver, and intestines.

In this situation, weight loss has a major effect and the use of Cholestin-3 can have an additional effect. In one middle-aged man treated at our center, diet and exercise lowered his cholesterol level from 300 mg/dL to 235 mg/dL over a period of about six weeks. He then began taking Cholestin-3, and experienced a further dip in his cholesterol level, from 235 mg/dL to 198 mg/dL. It is important not to expect dietary supplements to do too much in this situation. Read Chapters 5 and 7 carefully, and see your doctor regarding the importance of weight loss in your case.

FINE TUNING WHEN EVERYTHING IS NORMAL

We keep redefining the concept of "normal." When I was in college, the average cholesterol level in the United States was about 250. Just twenty years later, the average had dropped to 210. However, we now know that it is still possible for heart disease to occur with a cholesterol level as low as 180. Most prevention-oriented physicians recommend that their patients get their cholesterol levels below 200 to minimize the risk of heart disease. Recently, the desirable cholesterol levels have been set even lower, with some cardiologists suggesting that a cholesterol level of 150 is a more desirable goal.

I define fine tuning as seeking to become even healthier. You can never be too healthy. Most of the prevention benefit you get is from that first bit of prevention. Lowering your body weight to an ideal weight and increasing your daily exercise regimen provide real benefits. However, if you want to extend your life by reducing the progression of events that occur even in healthy people, then this information is for you.

Fine tuning is the process by which you attempt to retard the progression of atherosclerosis within your body's cells. To accomplish this end, you must counter-act several processes:

- The tendency for cholesterol particles to become oxi-dized and trapped in the walls of your blood vessels

- The tendency of the blood to form clots in areas af-fected by atherosclerosis

- The tendency to have high blood levels of homocys-teine, which can accelerate atherosclerosis

Table 11.1 provides a list of various fine-tuning sub-stances and their actions. While I can't provide you with specific dosages for all substances, I can provide some ranges. I can also give you some general advice. Read as much material as you can on natural supplements and products. Always carefully read the labels on any products you use. Start with low dosages and slowly work your way up. Also, talk to your doctor, especial-ly if you have a pre-existing condition of any kind.

Table 11.1. Fine-Tuning Substances

Active Substance	Natural Product	Supplement	Action	Daily Dosage
Acetylsalicylic acid	Willow tree bark	Aspirin	Anticoagulant	75–150 mg (baby aspirin)
Allicin	Garlic	Garlic pills	Lowers blood pressure cholesterol	One fresh clove or 600–900 mg powder
Cholestin-3	Red yeast	Cholestin-3 brand	Lowers cholesterol	2.4 mg
Eicosapentanoic acid	Fish	Fish oil caps	Anticoagulant	3 grams
Folic acid	Dark green vegetables	Folate pills	Lowers homocysteine	400 mcg
Niacin	Fish, poultry	Niacin pills	Lowers triglyceride	See package insert

There are also many different substances that have an-tioxidant activity (explained in Chapter 10). Some of these work directly as antioxidants, while others are involved in various steps of the atherosclerotic process that are less well understood. Our knowledge in this area is evolving. Natural medicines and a number of over-the-counter medications can both be used for these fine-tuning activities. For some antioxidants such as vitamin C and vitamin E, there are supplements available and their recommended dosages for antioxidant effects are known (see Chapter 10). For others, there are still no available supplements. Table 11.2 provides a list of the leading antioxidants.

Table 11.2. Leading Antioxidants

Antioxidant	Food Source	Supplement Source
Alpha tocopherol	Wheat germ	Vitamin E pills
Ascorbic acid	Citrus fruits	Vitamin C pills
Beta-carotene	Carrots	Beta-carotene pills
Cryptoxanthin	Fruits	No supplement
Lutein	Fruits	Lutein pills
Lycopene	Tomatoes	Lycopene-enriched food and pills
Monascorubrin	Red spice	*M. purpureus yeast* (Cholestin-3)
Polyphenols	Green tea	Green tea pills
OPC	Grape seeds, pine tree bark	OPC pills
Zeaxanthin	Fruits	No supplement

How far should you go with this fine-tuning activity? As long as you take care of the big picture with diet, exercise, and stress reduction, feel free to tinker as much as you like. Just don't take extremely large dosages of any substance without talking to your doctor first.

PUTTING YOUR KNOWLEDGE TO WORK

Knowledge is wonderful. It is fun to learn new things, but in the end it is only those things you do that really help you. To improve your lifestyle, you need to commit to making changes. Visualize where you want to be three months from now. If you would like to be exercising and fit, take the steps now to join a gym and schedule workouts three times a week. If you want to eat less fat and more fiber, change this week's shopping list and make better choices in restaurants. If you want to reduce stress, set aside some time for yourself. Read some light fiction. Take a Sunday to do nothing but enjoy life.

The week is the most practical unit of human behavior. Daily to-do lists just don't give you the complete picture. If you take your whole week and schedule your various activities by their importance in your life, you will be able to balance your priorities in health, fitness, and personal happiness. For instance, pick three days on which you plan to exercise. Write down when you plan to take your supplements and record your meals for one week. Be sure to give yourself at least one full day off, even if it is split between your weekend days and weekdays. See the sample schedule in Figure 11.1.

Once you have completed your calendar, you have defined your personal needs. Now comes your job and work responsibilities. Take the same calendar and add in the five most important things you must accomplish this week. Put them in your schedule when you are fresh and relaxed, not harried. How can you best relate your work to your personal responsibilities?

Notice that we are putting things in reverse of the usual order. You come first, then your job. This does not mean you work out every day and ignore your career. It does mean you pay yourself first, making sure

Mon.	Tues.	Wed.	Thurs.	Fri.	Sat.	Sun.
7am–Brkfst	Brkfst GYM	Brkfst	Brkfst GYM	Brkfst	Brkfst GYM	Sleep late DAY OFF
12 noon–Lunch	Lunch	Lunch	Lunch	Lunch	Lunch	Brunch
3pm–Snack	Snack	Snack	Snack	Snack	Snack	Snack
7pm–Dinner WALK	Dinner	Dinner WALK	Dinner	Dinner WALK	Dinner	Dinner

Figure 11.1. Sample Weekly Schedule

you have the health to enjoy your life. At work, be sure to have uninterrupted time when no one can enter your space each day. This is the time to get your most pressing work done. Try to develop a routine where the same types of tasks occur on the same days each week. That way your body can develop a biorhythm that is synchronized to the type of work being done each day. The more routine you can work into your job by compartmentalizing tasks and time, the more relaxed your life will become.

This cannot be done overnight. You must work at it over several months to put it into effect. The result will be a fuller, happier life. And you won't have to say, "I just can't find the time to exercise" anymore! This exercise program, along with your new diet and supplement regimens, will give you the piece of mind that comes with contributing to your own better health.

CHAPTER 12

Where Do We Go
From Here?

Because heart disease is the leading cause of death in this country, I feel that breakthroughs in the natural treatment of risk factors associated with heart disease can save the lives and improve the health of millions of people. As a doctor, I look forward to helping my patients lead better lives because of natural remedies. As a patient, you should look forward to sharing responsibility for your health with your health care provider by making the lifestyle changes needed to make natural remedies effective. However, heart disease and its related conditions are only a small part of the natural-medicine picture.

With each passing year, more and more people are discovering the power of natural substances. Natural medicine is now big business. According to a 1995 survey, the top ten herbal products accounted for 55 percent of the 1.27 billion dollar industry in natural products. The leading sellers were echinacea and garlic, with about 10 percent each. Goldenseal and ginseng had about 7 percent of the market. Gingko biloba, aloe vera, and saw palmetto each had about 4.5 percent. These products are being sold for a variety of purposes, as shown in Table 12.1.

Table 12.1. Natural Remedies and Their Uses

Product	Use
Aloe vera	Wound healing, immune defenses
Echinacea	Immune defenses
Garlic	Blood pressure and cholesterol lowering
Gingko biloba	Enhanced mental functioning
Ginseng	Enhanced energy
Goldenseal	Immune defenses
Saw palmetto	Prostate health

For many of these natural remedies, there is a tradition of use. Native Americans on the Great Plains used echinacea. It was so effective in reducing the duration of cold symptoms that it was sold in American drug stores until the 1950s. The Gingko biloba tree was said to have been saved from extinction in the Ice Age by the Chinese. It is an ancient and complex plant said to have originated some 250 million years ago. It has complex chemicals within it that have been extensively studied for their ability to enhance mental function. Saw palmetto contains substances that may help reduce prostate enlargement and may be able to inhibit the growth of prostate cancer cells. Aloe vera contains a substance called glucomannan, which may help wound healing.

These so-called folk remedies of the past are the basis for the natural medicines of the future. As more research examines the origins of these plants, we will no doubt discover new natural medicines that will benefit humankind.

There is now an office to promote research into dietary supplements, including natural remedies, at the National Institutes of Health called the Office of Dietary Supplements Research. This office encourages the study of natural dietary supplements through research of the type my colleagues and I are doing at UCLA with Cholestin-3. The best of the natural medicines must be tested in Western laboratories using modern concepts born of the technologies of cellular and molecular biology. Whenever possible, these dietary supplements should be tested using the double-blind, randomized prospective clinical trial, which keeps the investigators and the subjects from knowing who has the active substance and who has a placebo. In this way, the legitimate effects of the many natural remedies can be adequately tested and proven. Another need is for the standardization of measurement methods for different preparations.

However, you cannot rely solely on natural remedies to get the desired result. You need to take things into your own hands and do all of the natural things that should be done to aid the healing process. Throughout this book, I have stressed the need to put diet, exercise, and lifestyle in proper perspective relative to the cholesterol-lowering substances. This includes natural remedies such as Cholestin-3. By using natural remedies, you can treat ailments at an earlier stage to achieve true prevention. That has been the message of this book.

WHAT ABOUT OTHER NATURAL MEDICINES IN THE FUTURE?

The field of natural-medicine research has great possibilities as we rediscover the co-evolution of humans and plants on Earth. For example, we may soon have a natural contraceptive and a postmenopausal hormone replacement. In the year 600 B.C., on the Greek island of Cyrenea, there was a contraceptive based on a now extinct form of fennel. It worked simply by preventing the implantation of the fertilized egg in the uterus. It had no side effects. If this could be reproduced today, it would eliminate the side effects that occur in women who use oral contraceptives made with estrogen and progesterone.

The modern-day descendants of this fennel contain a class of compounds called isoflavones, which can interfere with the action of estrogens or act as weak estrogens. These substances are called phytoestrogens. Currently there are trade-offs with the estrogen or estrogen/progesterone pills and patches prescribed to women over fifty. They are said to reduce the risk of heart disease and osteoporosis, but may increase the risk of breast cancer. The use of isoflavones from plant sources could solve this problem.

Perhaps the greatest promise of the plant world for humankind would be an increase in the maximum lifespan. Studies carried out in rats and mice show that it is possible to extend maximum lifespan. In humans, the maximum recorded lifespan is about 120 years. In the experiments now repeated in many laboratories, an extension of lifespan in mice of up to 100 percent has been demonstrated. In humans, this would correspond to living between 160 and 240 years.

The key element in determining lifespan is the same process of oxidation that we discussed in Chapter 10 concerning cholesterol. This process occurs at measurable rates in all proteins and fats, as well as in RNA and DNA, the genetic-blueprint molecules in each cell. By using a variety of different antioxidants, it may be possible to slow this process. This has been demonstrated in animals, but not in humans.

The second potential area for exploration relates to an enzyme called telomerase. This enzyme restores DNA lost each time a cell replicates. A noncancer cell can only replicate about twenty times before it dies. Cancer cells, on the other hand, continue to reproduce themselves for years. Cancer cells have telomerase to restore the cell's DNA with each replication. The only normal cells in humans that have telomerase are certain intestinal cells, as well as one type of prostate-gland cell and the germ cells that give rise to sperm. Why is the telomerase enzyme distributed in this way? How is it regulated? Can any plant product modulate telomerase? These are questions that may hold the key to unlocking the mystery of aging.

NATURAL PRODUCTS THEN AND NOW

Natural products have a long history. They were born at the dawn of time, developed through hundreds of generations in prehistory, and brought to the land of Egypt. At the time of the Pharaohs there was a great body of knowledge on herbal medicine. Then, after the Romans destroyed the great library at Alexandria, this knowledge was lost. The knowledge reappeared in India with Ayurvedic medicine and made its way along the Silk Road to China, where camels carried the secrets of the ages. In China, the knowledge was committed to books. Again the ancient books were destroyed, so we are left with an imperfect oral tradition of traditional Chinese medicine.

In the Middle Ages, some of the herbal knowledge re-emerged. It is said that some of the women burned as witches in the 1600s were practicing herbal medicine. Until the middle of the twentieth century, pharmacy schools studied pharmacognosy, the study of herbs, and doctors studied herbal medicines. Then in the 1950s, this field of study was dropped from medical and pharmacy school curricula in the belief that the discovery of modern drugs would replace herbal medicine. Only now that we have the tools to study the relationship between humans and plants can we go back and find the real clues to curing heart disease, cancer, and other chronic diseases associated with aging.

We live at an exciting point in human history. After decades of turning our backs on the power of Nature, we are rediscovering the wonderful world of plant medicines that surrounds us. We have learned the benefits and drawbacks of the prescription drugs, and are now relegating them to their proper place in the treatment of disease.

The coming age will profoundly change our views about medicine. No longer will we just pop a pill and hope for the best. We are developing wholistic treatments that combine natural supplements with effective types of diet, exercise, and lifestyle changes. Together, we will learn how to make heart disease a thing of the past. We don't have all the answers yet, but the pieces of the puzzle are starting to fall into place. The knowledge we have gained in the past decade is truly remarkable, and new discoveries occur every day.

Yet we have learned so much already. This book has shown you the latest advances in natural medicine. Now is the time to put all this information to work for you. Develop your personal program for the prevention of heart disease, and implement it as soon as possible. Then you too can discover the natural way to a healthy heart.

References

Chapter 1
The New Path to a Healthy Heart

Kannel WB and Schatzkin A. Risk factor analysis. *Progress Cardiovasc Dis* 26:309, 1984.

Morrison JA, Nambodiri K, Green P, and others. Familial aggregation of lipids and lipoproteins in an early identification of dyslipoproteinemia: the Collaborative Lipid Research Clinics Family Study. *JAMA* 250:1860, 1983.

Ornish D, Brown S, Scherwitz LW, and others. Can lifestyle changes reverse coronary heart disease? *Lancet* 336:129, 1990.

Summary of the second report of the National Cholesterol Education Program (NCEP) expert panel on detection, evaluation, and treatment of high blood cholesterol in adults. (Adult Treatment Panel II) *JAMA* 269:3015–3023, 1993.

Chapter 2
The Nature of the Human Heart

Blankenhorn DH, Nessim SA, Johnson RL, and others. Beneficial effects of combined colestipol-niacin therapy on coronary atherosclerosis and coronary venous bypass grafts. *JAMA* 257:3233, 1987.

Crouse JR. Gender, lipoproteins, diet and cardiovascular risk. *Lancet* 1:318, 1989.

Falk E and others. Coronary plaque disruption. *Circulation* 92:657, 1995.

Goode GK and Heagerty AM. *In vitro* responses of human peripheral small arteries in hypercholesterolemia and effects of therapy. *Circulation* 91:2898, 1995.

Lipid Research Clinics Program. The Lipid Research Clinics Coronary Primary Prevention Trial Results, II: relationship of reduction in incidence of coronary heart disease to cholesterol lowering. *JAMA* 251:355, 1984.

Chapter 3
Lessons From Around the World:
Risk Factors for Heart Disease

Multiple Risk Factor Intervention Trial Research Group. Multiple Risk Factor Trial, risk factor changes and mortality. *JAMA* 248:1465, 1982.

Reaven GM. Looking at the world through LDL-cholesterol glasses. *J Nutrition* 116:1143, 1986.

Stamler J, Wentworth D, and Neaton JD. Is relationship between serum cholesterol and risk of premature death from coronary heart disease continuous or graded? Findings in 356,222 primary screenees of the MRFIT. *JAMA* 256:2823, 1986.

Chapter 4
The Cholesterol Thermostat

Brown MS and Goldstein JL. A receptor-mediated pathway for cholesterol homeostasis. *Science* 232:34, 1986.

Brunzell JD and Austin MA. Plasma triglyceride levels and coronary heart disease. *New Engl J Med* 320:1273, 1989.

Castelli WP. The triglyceride issue: a view from Framingham. *Am Heart J* 112:432, 1986.

Fredrickson DS, Levy RI, and Lees RS. Fat transport in lipoproteins—an integrated approach to mechanisms and disorders. *New Engl J Med* 85:447, 1976.

Chapter 5
Eat to Your Heart's Content:
The Skinny on Lowering Cholesterol Levels

Grundy SM. Comparison of monounsaturated fatty acids and carbohydrates for lowering plasma cholesterol. *New Engl J Med* 314:745, 1986.

Kris-Etherton PM (ed). *Cardiovascular Disease: Nutrition for Prevention and Treatment.* Chicago: The American Dietetic Association, 1990.

Pritikin N. *The Pritikin Program for Diet and Exercise.* New York: Grosset and Dunlap, 1982.

Rimm EB, Ascherio A, and Giovanucei E. Vegetable, fruit, and cereal fiber intake and risk of coronary heart disease among men. *JAMA* 275:447–451, 1996.

Chapter 6
Stress and Your Heart: The Mind-Body Connection

Friedman M, Thoresen CE, Gill JJ, and others. Alteration

of Type A behavior and reduction in cardiac recurrences in myocardial infarction. *Am Heart J* 108:237, 1984.

Haynes SG, Feinleib M, and Kannel WB. The relationship of psychological factors to coronary heart disease. *Am J Epidemiol* 111:37, 1980.

Klatsky AI and others. Risk of cardiovascular mortality in alcohol drinkers, ex-drinkers, and non-drinkers. *Am J Cardiology* 66:1237, 1990.

Ornish D. *Stress, Diet and Your Heart.* New York: Holt, Rinehart and Winston, 1982.

Chapter 7
What to Do When You Feel the Urge to Exercise

Blair SN, Haskell WL, Ho P, and others. Assessment of habitual physical activity by a seven day recall in a community survey and controlled experiments. *Am J Epidemiol* 122:794, 1985.

Paffenbarger RS and Hale WE. Work activity and coronary heart mortality. *New Engl J Med* 292:545, 1975.

Tran ZV, Weltiman A, Glass GV, and others. The effects of exercise on blood lipids and lipoproteins: a meta-analysis of studies. *Med Sci Sports Exer* 15:393, 1983.

Chapter 8
Are Drugs the Answer?

Blankenhorn DH, Azen SP, and Kramsch DH. Coronary angiographic changes with lovastatin therapy. The monitored atherosclerosis regression study (MARS). *Ann Intern Med* 119:969–976, 1993.

Carlson LA and Rosenhamer G. Reduction of mortality

in the Stockholm Ischemic Heart Disease Secondary Prevention Study by combined treatment with clofibrate and nicotinic acid. *Acta Med Scand* 223:405, 1988.

LaRosa JC. Cholesterol-lowering and the cost-effective prevention of recurrent heart disease. *Cardiovascular Reviews and Reports* 17(8):10–28, 1996.

National Cholesterol Education Program Expert Panel. Report on detection, evaluation, and treatment of high blood cholesterol in adults. *Arch Intern Med* 148:36, 1988.

Scandinavian Simvastatin Survival Study Group. Randomised trial of cholesterol lowering in 4444 patients with coronary heart disease: the Scandinavian Simvastatin survival study (4S). *Lancet* 344:1383–1389, 1994.

Shepherd J, Cobbe SM, Ford I, and others. Prevention of coronary heart disease with pravastatin in men with hypercholesterolemia. *New Engl J Med* 333:1301–1307, 1995.

Chapter 9
Cholesterol Reduction and the East-West Connection

Endo A. Monacolin K, a new hypocholesterolemic agent produced by a *Monascus* species. *J Antibiotics* 32:852, 1979.

Li CL, Li YF, and Hou ZL. Xuezhikang toxicity study. *Bull China Pharmacol Soc* 12:12, 1995.

Shen Z, Yu P, Sun M, Chi J, Zhou Y, Zhu X, Yang C, and He C. A prospective study on ZhiTai capsule in the treatment of primary hyperlipidemia. *Natl Med J China* 76:156–157, 1996.

Shuyun X, Rulian B, and Xiu C. *Pharmacology Experiment Methodology*. Second Edition. Beijing: People's Health Press, 1991, p. 1047.

Wang J, Su M, Lu Z, Kou W, Chi J, Yu P, and Wang W. Clinical trial of extract of *Monascus purpureus* (red yeast) in the treatment of hyperlipidemia. *Chin J Exp Therapeutics for Prepared Chinese Medicine* 12:1–5, 1995.

Zhu Y, Li CL, and Wang YY. Effects of Xuezhikang on blood lipids and lipoprotein concentrations of rabbits and quails with hyperlipidemia. *Chinese J Pharmacol* 30: 4–8, 1995.

Zhu Y, Li CL, Wang YY, Zhu JS, Chang J, and Kritchevsky D. *Monascus purpureus* (red yeast): a natural product that lowers blood cholesterol in animal models of hypercholesterolemia. Manuscript submitted to *Nutrition Research*.

Chapter 10
Other Natural Medicines

Anderson JW. *The HCF Exchanges: The High Carbohydrate-High Fiber (HCF) Nutrition Plan.* Lexington KY: HCF Diabetes Foundation, 1987.

Anderson JW, Johnstone BM, and Cook-Newell ME. Meta-analysis of the effects of soy protein intake on serum lipids. *New Engl J Med* 333:276–282, 1995.

Anthony MS, Clarkson TB, Hughes CL, Morgan TM, and Burke GL. Soybean isoflavones improve cardiovascular risk factors without affecting the reproductive system of prepubertal rhesus monkeys. *J Nutrition* 126:43–50, 1996.

Beynen AC. Comparison of the mechanisms proposed to explain the hypocholesterolemic effect of soy protein versus casein in experimental animals. *J Nutr Sci Vitaminol* 36:587–593, 1990.

Carlson LA and others. Pronounced lowering of serum levels of lipoprotein Lp(a) in hyperlipidemic subjects treated with nicotinic acid. *Arch Int Med* 226:271, 1989.

Denke MA. Lack of efficacy of low-dose sitostanol therapy as an adjunct to a cholesterol-lowering diet in men with moderate hypercholesterolemia. *Am J Clin Nutr* 61: 392, 1995.

Fulder S. *The Garlic Book.* Garden City Park NY: Avery Publishing Group, 1997.

Koval GM. Dietary oat fiber sources and blood lipids. *JAMA* 268:985, 1992.

Mattson FH and others. Optmizing the effects plant sterols on cholesterol absorption in man. *Am J Clin Nutrition* 35:697, 1982.

Nordoy A and others. Individual effects of saturated fatty acids and fish oil on plasma lipids and lipoproteins in normal men. *Am J Clin Nutrition* 57:634, 1993.

Rimm EB and others. Vitamin E consumption and the risk of coronary heart disease in men. *New Engl J Med* 337:1, 1993.

Rudin D and Felix C. *Omega 3 Oils.* Garden City Park NY: Avery Publishing Group, 1996.

Stampfer MJ and Malinow RM. Can lowering homocysteine levels reduce cardiovascular risk? *New Engl J Med* 332:328, 1995.

Stampfer MJ and others. Vitamin E consumption and the risk of coronary heart disease in women. *New Engl J Med* 20:1444, 1993.

Warshafsky S and others. Effect of garlic on total serum cholesterol. *Annals Intern Med* 119:599, 1993.

Chapter 11
Putting It All Together

Kannel WB. Lipids, diabetes, and coronary heart disease: insights from the Framingham Study. *Am Heart J* 110: 1100, 1985.

NIH Consensus Conference. Triglyceride, high-density lipoprotein, and coronary heart disease. *JAMA* 269:505, 1993.

Pearson T and others. Optimal risk factor management in the patient after coronary revascularization. *Circulation* 90:3125, 1994.

Rifkind BM and Segal P. Lipid Research Clinics program reference values for hyperlipidemia and hypolipidemia. *JAMA* 250:1869, 1983.

Glossary

Italicized words are defined elsewhere in the Glossary.

Acetylcholine. A chemical that, under normal conditions, causes a blood vessel to dilate. However, if the vessel's *endothelium* is injured, or if there is too much *cholesterol* in the bloodstream, acetylcholine will cause the vessel to constrict.

Aerobic training. Exercises done primarily to strengthen the heart, such as running and cycling.

Angina. Chest pain that occurs because of inadequate blood flow to the heart.

Antioxidants. Substances that can neutralize *free radicals*, which helps prevent the *oxidation* of *cholesterol*.

Aorta. The largest artery in the body. It carries blood from the heart to the rest of the body.

Apolipoproteins. Proteins carried by *lipoproteins* that enable the lipoproteins to attach to *receptors* on the body's cells. Once this attachment occurs, a lipoprotein can deliver its *cholesterol* and *triglycerides* to the cell.

Aspirin. A naturally derived drug that reduces blood *viscosity*.

Atherosclerosis. The process by which *oxidized cholesterol* forms *plaques* on the walls of arteries, causing the arteries to become narrowed and stiff. A *heart attack* or stroke can occur if a clot becomes stuck in the narrowed artery, stopping the flow of blood.

Atorvastatin. A drug that acts as an *HMG-CoA reductase inhibitor*.

Atromid-S. The brand name of *clofibrate*, a *fibrate*.

Beta-carotene. A precursor of vitamin A that acts as an *antioxidant*.

Bile acids. Substances that help the body digest fats. Bile acids are produced by the liver from *cholesterol*.

Bile-acid sequestrants. Drugs that soak up *cholesterol-*laden *bile acids* within the intestines in order to remove them from the body.

Blood pressure. A measure of the resistance to blood flow in the capillaries. High blood pressure can damage the circulatory system, leading to heart disease or stroke.

Burnout depression. Depression that results from unrelenting stress.

Catecholamines. Hormones that trigger the body's stress

response, which includes a racing pulse and a rise in *blood pressure.*

CBS disease. See *cystathione beta synthase deficiency.*

Cholesterol. A white, flaky substance that has many important functions throughout the body, especially in the creation and maintenance of cell membranes. Cholesterol must be packaged together with *triglycerides* to create *lipoproteins* before it can be carried through the bloodstream. Cholesterol only becomes a problem if it gathers on the walls of arteries and is *oxidized.*

Cholesterol thermostat. The genetically predetermined levels of blood *cholesterol* that the body attempts to maintain. This mechanism, which evolved at a time when the human diet was deficient in cholesterol and fat, can cause the amount of blood cholesterol to rise to dangerous levels among sedentary people who eat high-fat diets.

Cholestin-3. An American food supplement prepared from *Hong qu* that can help lower blood cholesterol levels when used as part of a regimen of diet, exercise, and stress reduction.

Cholestyramine. A drug that acts as a *bile-acid sequestrant.*

Chylomicrons. Molecules that carry *cholesterol* from the intestines into the bloodstream.

Clofibrate. A drug that acts as a *fibrate.* It is not often used any more.

Co-evolution. The process by which plants and humans

have evolved together, with the human body adapting to substances present in plants.

Colestid. The brand name of *colestipol,* a *bile-acid sequestrant.*

Colestipol. A drug that acts as a *bile-acid sequestrant.*

Collateral blood vessels. Blood vessels that develop when a clot shuts down a *coronary artery* in order to carry blood around the affected area.

Coronary arteries. The arteries that carry blood to the heart itself.

Coronary artery disease. The development of *atherosclerosis* within the *coronary arteries.* Such disease narrows the arteries and increases the risk of *heart attack.*

Coronary calcification. The development of bone tissue that occurs within *plaques.*

Cystathione beta synthase deficiency (CBS disease). A rare genetic disorder that often leads to early heart disease. Individuals with CBS disease often have high blood levels of *homocysteine.*

Dietary cholesterol. See *exogenous cholesterol.*

Dysthymia. A form of mild depression seen in many people who are overweight.

EKG. See *electrocardiogram.*

Electrocardiogram (EKG). A graphic record of the heart muscle's electrical activity.

Endogenous cholesterol. *Cholesterol* that is produced by the body itself.

Endorphins. Morphinelike brain chemicals that promote a sense of calm and well-being. Endorphins are released during exercise.

Endothelium. The tissue that lines the inside of the blood vessels. *Atherosclerosis* of the endothelium lining the *coronary arteries* is called *coronary artery disease.*

Essential fatty acids. Fatty acids, includes the *omega-3 fatty acids*, that must be obtained from food. About 5 percent of each day's calories must come from fat in order to obtain required amounts of the essential fatty acids.

Exogenous cholesterol (dietary cholesterol). *Cholesterol* that comes from food.

Fatty-food intolerance. The stomach upset, diarrhea, and gas formation experienced by people who are used to a low-fat diet when they eat a high-fat food.

Fiber. See *insoluble fiber* and *water-soluble fiber.*

Fibrates. Drugs that reduce the production of *very-low-density lipoproteins* in the liver, which has the effect of lowering levels of *low-density lipoproteins* in the blood.

Fibrinogen. A protein that helps determine how readily the blood will clot.

Fluvastatin. A drug that acts as an *HMG-CoA reductase inhibitor.*

Foam cells. Cells that enter the artery wall to eat up

low-density lipoproteins that have been affected by *oxidation*. Once the foam cells do so, they also become trapped in the artery wall.

Free radicals. Substances that are produced during the body's processing of oxygen. Free radicals are unstable and can cause the *oxidation* of *cholesterol*.

Garlic. A plant food and traditional medicine that can reduce both *cholesterol* and *triglyceride* levels, promote *antioxidant* activity, and reduce blood *viscosity*.

Gemfibrozil. A drug that acts as a *fibrate*.

HDL. See *high-density lipoprotein*.

Heart attack. A condition in which a *coronary artery* becomes blocked by a clot, leading to the death of a section of heart tissue.

High-density lipoprotein (HDL). The "good" *cholesterol* that carries *low-density lipoproteins* back to the liver before the latter can settle in the artery walls and cause *plaques* to develop.

HMG-CoA reductase. An enzyme in the liver that stimulates the production of *cholesterol*.

HMG-CoA reductase inhibitors (statins). Drugs that inhibit the action of *HMG CoA reductase*, a liver chemical that stimulates *cholesterol* production.

Homeostasis. The body's tendency to maintain blood *cholesterol* at genetically predetermined levels.

Homocysteine. An amino acid that circulates in the

bloodstream. Individuals with high levels of homocysteine have an increased risk of developing *atherosclerosis* and heart disease.

Hong qu. A yeast used in China to create a food preservative and colorant. Certain strains contain *cholesterol*-inhibiting factors.

Insoluble fiber (roughage). Fiber that largely passes undigested through the intestines. It adds bulk to the stool and helps to clean off the intestinal walls. It does not affect *cholesterol* levels.

LDL. See *low-density lipoprotein*.

Lescol. The brand name of *fluvastatin*, an *HMG-CoA reductase inhibitor*.

Lipitor. The brand name of *atorvastatin*, an *HMG-CoA reductase inhibitor*.

Lipoprotein lipase. An enzyme that moves *triglycerides* from the bloodstream into the body's cells. This lowers the concentration of triglycerides in the bloodstream. The effects of lipoprotein lipase are enhanced by exercise.

Lipoproteins. Fat-and-protein packages that carry *cholesterol* and *triglycerides* through the bloodstream.

Lopid. The brand name of *gemfibrozil*, a *fibrate*.

Lorelco. The brand name of *probucol*.

Lovastatin. A drug that acts as an *HMG-CoA reductase inhibitor*.

Low-density lipoprotein (LDL). The "bad" *cholesterol* that can settle in the artery walls and cause *plaques* to develop.

Mevacor. The brand name of *lovastatin*, an *HMG-CoA reductase inhibitor*.

Mixed hyperlipidemia. A condition marked by high levels of *cholesterol* and *triglycerides*, with no genetic *low-density lipoprotein* defects present. It is often accompanied by obesity and diabetes.

Niacin. A B vitamin that can reduce both *cholesterol* and *triglyceride* levels, and stimulate the formation of *prostaglandins*.

Niacin flush. A totally harmless reddening and tingling of the skin experienced by some people when they take *niacin*. It tends to be a problem that goes away when one's body gets used to increased niacin levels.

Niacinamide. A substance formed in the liver from *niacin*. It can, like niacin, help prevent pellagra, a niacin-deficiency disease. However, niacinamide cannot affect *cholesterol* levels.

Omega-3 fatty acids. One of the two classes of *essential fatty acids*, and one that is most lacking in the modern diet. The omega-3s can lower levels of both *cholesterol* and *triglycerides*, and reduce blood *viscosity*.

Oxidation. The process by which *free radicals* cause various kinds of damage within the body. The oxidation of *cholesterol* is part of the process of *atherosclerosis*.

Phytosterols (sterols). Plant substances that are chemically related to *cholesterol*, and can compete with cholesterol for absorption through the intestinal wall. This helps to reduce blood cholesterol levels.

Plaques. *Cholesterol*-laden deposits on the inside surface of artery walls that develop as the result of *athero-sclerosis*.

Platelets. Small cells in the bloodstream that cause the blood to clot.

Potency. A drug's ability to do what it is designed to do, such as lower *cholesterol* levels.

Pravachol. The brand name of *pravastatin*, an *HMG-CoA reductase inhibitor*.

Pravastatin. A drug that acts as an *HMG-CoA reductase inhibitor*.

Probucol. A drug that inhibits the *oxidation* of *low-den-sity lipoproteins*. This helps to keep the LDLs from settling into the artery walls.

Pro-oxidants. Substances that encourage *oxidation*. Pro-oxidants come from many sources, including tobacco smoke and environmental pollution.

Prostaglandins. Chemicals that are involved in a wide variety of body functions, including the maintenance of healthy blood vessels.

Questran, Questran Light. Brand names for *cholestyra-mine*, a *bile-acid sequestrant*.

Receptors. Molecules on the cells of various organs that serve as attachment points for *apolipoproteins*. This allows *cholesterol* and *triglycerides* to be delivered to the cells.

Resistance training. Exercises done primarily to build the muscles, such as weightlifting.

Risk factors. Factors that determine one's risk of developing heart disease. These factors include genetic tendencies, diet, exercise level, stress level, body weight, *blood pressure,* presence of diabetes, use of tobacco and alcohol, and blood *cholesterol* level.

Roughage. See *insoluble fiber*.

Simvastatin. A drug that acts as an *HMG-CoA reductase inhibitor*.

Sitosterol. The most prevalent of the *phytosterols*. It is almost chemically identical to *cholesterol*.

Statins. See *HMG-CoA reductase inhibitors*.

Sterols. See *phytosterols*.

Target heart rate. The heart rate during *aerobic training* that causes the heart muscle to become stronger.

Total cholesterol. The total amount of cholesterol carried on the *HDL, LDL,* and *VLDL* particles in the blood.

Triglycerides. Fats that are the body's preferred form of energy storage. Triglycerides must be packaged together with *cholesterol* to create *lipoproteins* before they can be carried through the bloodstream.

Unconscious nervous system. The part of the nervous system that controls all functions not under conscious control, including heartbeat. Also called the autonomic nervous system.

Very-low-density lipoprotein (VLDL). A large *lipoprotein* that carries *cholesterol* and *triglycerides* through the bloodstream to the various tissues.

Viscosity. The thickness of a fluid. Increased blood viscosity can lead to the development of blood clots.

Vitamin C. A water-souble vitamin that acts as an *antioxidant*.

Vitamin E. A fat-souble vitamin that acts as an *antioxidant*.

VLDL. See *very-low-density lipoprotein*.

VLDL remnant. A *very-low-density lipoprotein* that has lost most of its *triglycerides*.

Water-soluble fiber. Fiber than can dissolve in water. In the intestines, it absorbs *cholesterol*-laden *bile acids* and carries them out of the body. This helps to reduce cholesterol levels in the bloodstream.

Xuezhikang. A Chinese extract prepared from *Hong qu* that can help lower blood *cholesterol* levels.

Zhitai. A Chinese extract prepared from *Hong qu* that can help lower blood *cholesterol* levels.

Zocor. The brand name of *simvastatin*, an *HMG-CoA reductase inhibitor*.

Index